Get In Shape Fast

SOCIAVERSE PUBLISHING

ISBN-13: 978-1516853601

ISBN-10: 1516853601

DEDICATION

This book is dedicated to all of the incredible professionals and companies who took the time to submit content to this book. It has been a pleasure working with each of you on the production of this book. The time you have all taken and the high-quality content that you have all shared has truly gone above and beyond anything we could have ever expected when we first set out to publish this book. Thank you to everyone who made this possible.

CONTENTS

DEDICATION..iii

CONTENTS...v

ACKNOWLEDGMENTS.......................................vii

INTRODUCTION..1

CHAPTER 1: HOPE COWGILL................................3

CHAPTER 2: ALEXANDRA ALLRED.........................13

CHAPTER 3: BRIAN STERLING-VETE......................35

CHAPTER 4: DR RICHARD E. HARRIS II &
    KEEON RUDDER...............................45

CHAPTER 5: ALEX PERRY..................................51

CHAPTER 6: BRANDON ROBERTS........................57

CHAPTER 7: HENRY HALSE...............................65

CHAPTER 8: ERIK CLINE..................................75

CHAPTER 9: TREVA BRANDON SCHARF...............81

CHAPTER 10: MARIE DELCIOPPO & LAUREN
    MANISCALCO.................................85

CHAPTER 11: MARISA SILVER.............................95

CHAPTER 12: ILARIA CAVAGNA.........................103

CHAPTER 13: CLIFFORD JOSEPH.......................115

CONCLUSION...131

ACKNOWLEDGMENTS

I'd like to thank the top Fitness coaches in America whose contributions of time and effort have made this book possible:

Hope Cowgill of inBalance

Alexandra Allred of Main Street Gym

Brian Sterling-Vete of MajorVision

Dr Richard E. Harris & Keeon Rudder of Von Elijah Fitness

Alex Parry of Character Strength & Conditioning

Brandon Roberts of Brandon's Blueprint

Henry Halse of Halse Strength & Fitness

Erik Cline of Erik Cline, Life Coach

Treva Brandon Scharf of Equinox

Marie Delcioppo of Lush Vitality

Lauren Maniscalco of Coastal Body Studio

Marisa Silver of In The Zone Personal Fitness

Ilaria Cavagna of Ilaria Cavagna, Fitness Trainer

Clifford Joseph of Fitness Essentials

I would also like to thank the hardworking staff of SociaVerse Publishing, who continue to change lives through the power of print.

INTRODUCTION

Have you ever had to get ready for an upcoming event only to realize that you are terribly out of shape?

Maybe it's an alumni gathering and the thought of your old friends seeing you with a beer belly or flabby arms terrify you. Maybe it's an upcoming wedding shoot and you can't bear the thought of paying tremendous sums of money of a less than ideal image of yourself and your spouse to be.

What's more, time is short and you wonder, "is there anything that you can do?"

The good news is that this book was written for you! We have approached some of the top fitness coaches in America with different backgrounds and areas of expertise to give you professional advice on what you can do.

What they share are based on years of experience working with different clients. Learn from them and use the gems contained in these pages to help you reach your fitness goals.

CHAPTER 1

HOPE COWGILL

Please tell us about your company here:

I am the owner of inBalance, a fitness studio in San Antonio, Texas. We provide all levels of yoga, Pilates, barre, cardio, and other fitness classes.

At inBalance you can find balance in life - for we not only teach Yoga, Pilates, Barre and invigorating Cardio classes, we also provide a sense of community for our members and help them achieve personal growth. What's more, our smaller classes mean they always get personal attention and beginners are always welcomed with open arms. We make sure that from day one, we know our student's name and fitness goals, so we help them get the results they want.

I have had a passion for rhythm and movement since I could walk and danced my way through high school and on my college dance team before discovering the benefits of Pilates and the mindfulness of yoga. After a decade of teaching fitness and earning countless certifications, I opened inBalance to help others enjoy the exhilaration of dance and the peace-of-mind that true health brings. In our welcoming, peaceful space everyone will be sure to discover new passions. And It doesn't matter how out of shape you feel you are, my studio is for everyone.

1. What is the best way to lose fat?

This is the question of the ages and has a much more complicated answer than most people want to know. To lose fat one must also build muscle. The more pounds of muscle, the fewer pounds of fat you have, and the more muscle, the more calories you burn without even trying! As you build muscle, you will burn fat. And there is no better way to build muscle than with strength training. Many people (namely women) are afraid of lifting weights, thinking they will get 'bulky'; but unless you are eating like a bodybuilder (who eats thousands and thousands of calories a day) there is no way you are going to get bulky. Strength training is what will build muscle, which in turn will burn fat. You don't necessarily have to be lifting hundreds of pounds; just adding a mix of light weight training will help build muscle. Simply doing cardio is not enough to lose fat; yes, it can help shed pounds but at some point, too much cardio will lead to losing muscle, which are not the pounds you want to be losing. Doing this will eventually slow down your metabolism and will have the opposite effect of what you are trying to do.

In addition to adding weights to your workout regime, it must also be followed by the right diet. Eating the right balance of carbs, protein, and fats, as well as adequate calories, is key to shedding fat. Not eating enough calories will leave your metabolism lagging, but eating too much of the wrong calories will leave you in a rut. The recommended balance of macro nutrients (carbs, fat, and protein) is around (depending on who you ask) 40% carbs, 30% protein and 30% fat. Keeping your calories as close to this balance as possible will kick start your fat loss and keep your energy at all time highs!

Mixing in strength training sessions, whether that is simply lifting weights, trying interval strength classes, Crossfit, or some other form of strength training, with the proper diet, this is sure to help lose fat and build muscle keeping that metabolism revved up.

2. I have an event coming up in 2 months. What's my best strategy for getting in better shape by then?

I am not a believer in 'quick fixes' as far as fitness and health are concerned, but for those looking to get in shape fast, there are some things to be done to look and feel your best. The first tip I always give my clients always goes back to diet. Diet accounts for 75-80% of your weight loss goals and you should always place the most emphasis on what is going in your mouth!

Cutting out sugar, especially refined sugar and alcohol, will allow you to lose any bloat and keep skin clear while also allowing you to kick start your weight loss. Your diet should rely mostly on green veggies and protein during this prep time. Also, stay hydrated! This will help flush out toxins and keep you full longer. Thirst is often misinterpreted as hunger, so stay hydrated to keep those signals from getting mixed up.

As far as exercise, quick, high-intensity workouts will really rev up your metabolism and burn fat. Think High-Intensity Interval Training (HIIT); those exercises that are short and intense, that get your heart rate up FAST. These are workouts that will allow you to keep burning fat well after the workout is over. And of course, don't forget to replenish your muscles after your workouts! A healthy blend of protein and carbs, ideally a 2: 1 carbs to protein ration, will rebuild muscles and keep your metabolism going.

3. Is walking or running better for fat loss?

The answer to this all depends on intensity, as well as if you are looking for quicker results or looking at a long term plan.

Walking might be a better long-term plan for fat-burning when it comes to those who overweight. Low-intensity exercise, like walking, rely more heavily on fat reserves than calorie reserves (using a higher percentage of fat callers for energy) for completion, making this an effective way to target fat-burning. However, low to moderate exercise doesn't burn fat as quickly as high-intensity workouts. It's possible to amp up fat-burning and calorie-burning for walkers by adding intervals, such as hills or adding plyometrics, like squats, lunges or high knees.

So whether you are walking or running, in order to burn fat, you should include intervals. When you make your body work harder by adding intervals, it has to work harder to get more oxygen, so now your body is now working less efficiently; it has to burn more calories to do the activity (running or walking). In addition, high-intensity intervals will rev up your metabolism so that you will continue that calorie burn well after you have finished working out (that 'after-burn' everyone is looking for!). This will help boost your metabolism, which will increase those fat burning hormones. Over the long run, this will equate to a larger percentage of fat loss, more so than steady state cardio at a moderate intensity level. Because, whether you are using fat or carbs are being as fuel, what matters most is how many total calories you burn for the time you have exercised. Shorter, more intense intervals are key to burning fat.

4. Should I do cardio or weight training?

There is no either-or answer to this question; you must do both! As stated in my answer to the first question, strength (or weight) training is key to building muscle which helps burn fat. Weight training also helps increase bone density, reduces stress and cholesterol, and can be viewed as a functional type of training, meaning that building strength helps you in other aspects of life. Lifting heavy objects, carrying kids, or just walking up the stairs are done with ease once you have built strength from your weight training regime. Adding a cardio element to this will help keep your metabolism working and round out your training. Keeping your heart healthy is just as important as the rest of your body. Plus, mixing the 2 (cardio and weights) in an interval workout is the best way to burn fat so it's a win/win!

5. What are your recommended workouts for fast results?

High-Intensity Interval Training (HIIT) is the best workout for fast results. These are quick high-intensity workouts that get your heart rate up quickly, allows short spurts of rest, then on to another interval. Because these workouts put you in the aerobic state (when you are working hard and feel like you're out of breath) this really spikes your metabolism, not burning calories, but burning fat, and you continue to burn after your workout is over. Not only are you getting a cardiovascular workout, but you are also getting strength training, trying to get in as many reps as you can during those intervals.

Another way to get fast results is to try something new! Tricking the body and making it try something it has never done before (or has not done in a long time) will always lend fast results. Eventually, your body adapts, so it is always good to change up your workout periodically, trying something new or adding a new aspect to your training.

6. How can I speed up my recovery period?

Post workout nutrition is key. After a workout is important to replenish with a snack that is a 2: 1 ration of carbs to protein.

This combo will help rebuild what you've broken down during a workout. Staying hydrated is another important part of recovery. Working muscles need hydration, and they also need hydration to recover and prepare them for the next workout. Getting an adequate amount of sleep each night is also important to recovery. Sleep is the time when the body recovers; when you skimp out on this, your body will let you know. Your workouts will suffer, your brain function will suffer, and your body will start to break down.

7. How often should I workout?

This question depends on what your goals are. If it is maintenance, working out at least 45 minutes a day 4-5 days a week is ample. If you are looking to lose weight, you would need to amp it up; adding another day of training and making your sessions a bit longer or adding intensity to shorter workouts.

8. How do I get a flat stomach?

The next 2 questions can be answered together...first, it is important to know there is no way to spot reduce fat. When you lose fat, you do not get to choose where it comes from! You just have to work on overall fat loss and then building muscle in its place. Getting a 'flat stomach' means you are looking to get rid of belly fat. If this is your goal, there are few things to look at. First, take a look at your diet. If it consists off too much alcohol and sugar (especially refined sugars) this should be your first step. Cleaning up your diet can have a huge impact on your waistline! After cleaning up your diet, take a look at your workouts. Are you adding some days of high-intensity? Are you adding some exercises that require you to use your whole body as resistance (think planks, push ups, plyometric type exercises)? These are ways to shed fat and build your core, working your abs from all directions. A consistent practice of all of these factors will help push you towards your goal of a flat tummy.

9. How do I get rid of flabby arms?

I repeat, there is no way to 'spot reduce'. Following the first couple steps listed in #9 will allow for fat loss. After you've cleaned your diet and added high-intensity workouts to burn fat, you need to focus on steering training to ad muscle to lose 'flab' on those arms. Losing weight alone won't do it; you must build muscle there that replaces the fat! Adding weight training, working every part of the arm (biceps, triceps, shoulders, deltoids) will help add muscle and arms will look more tone, less flabby.

10. What short workouts can I do between work?

There is a ton of options for quick workouts throughout the day. Taking a walk arounds the building, jogging laps through the parking lot, running or just walking the stairs is a great workout! There are also many many executrices that can be done at your desk, just using your desk and chair. YouTube has exercises, as well as our Instagram and Facebook page! Exercise for arms, legs, abs, the possibilities are endless! Really there is no excuse for 'not having the time' at workout at work.

11. What is the best diet to follow?

This is a somewhat loaded question...and depending on who you ask you will get a MILLION different answers. I don't really believe in high-restriction diets, those that restrict certain foods or food groups, unless it is a dietary need (I for one am lactose intolerant so dairy is out of the question!) or a personal choice (those that choose not to eat meat for ethical reason). I believe in BALANCE; a balanced diet is a healthy diet. A balanced diet is also the key to keeping your weight under control. As I stated in a previous question, a balanced diet should follow the 40/30/30 ratio: 40% carbs, 30% protein, 30% fat. This diet should be full of bright colored veggies and fruits, hormone and antibiotic free protein, and healthy fats, and limit the intake of processed food. Whole foods are key! With this ratio, you should also be sure to stay nourished through the day, eating snacks or several small meals throughout the day. Once you let your blood sugar get too low by staying hungry for hours, you allow your insulin level to spike, sending your body into that starvation mode which tells your body to hang on to body fat for storage because it needs nourishment...this is bad! Eating every 3 or 4 hours is key to keeping your hormone levels at sufficient levels to keep your insulin levels stable.

12. Do I need to take dietary supplements?

This is really a question of personal preference. If you are eating a diet that contains adequate nutrients, as well as sufficient fruits and vegetables, you should be getting the right amount of vitamins and minerals. However those on special diets or who are extremely active probably need to supplement certain nutrients, like B vitamins. Women should also stay with a regular calcium/vitamin D supplement to keep osteoporosis at bay. I am also a believer in taking a glucosamine supplement for those who are active to protect joints.

13. What tips do you have for healthy food on the go?

As mentioned previously, whole foods are key, so if you need to go snacks, go for things like fruit, nuts, trail mix or homemade energy bars. Be careful with energy bars sold in stores; many of them have many added sugars and can de-rail your day as far as nutrition goes. I love to make homemade energy bars, because you can play around with ingredients, adding different fruits and nuts, and even adding protein powder so you can get all your macro nutrients in one snack!

14. Who is your ideal client to work with?

One who is self-motivated! You can only push a person so hard and if they do not have the drive from the inside, they give up quickly and work to a point where they will not be pushed. This usually turns into frustration and can have a terrible effect on their workouts and their progress. Someone who is self-motivated comes in ready to work hard and loves to be pushed.

15. What are the main benefits of working with a personal trainer?

Getting that one on one attention is a great way to set clear goals and track your progress. Working with a training established more accountability; you become accountable for your workouts to your trainer; someone who expects you to show up pushes you and won't let you cheat on your workouts! Insert chapter one text here. Insert chapter one text here.

Please tell us how readers can get in contact with you here:

Our website: inbalancesanantonio.com

Email me at hope@inbalancesanantonio.com

Follow us on Facebook, Instagram and Twitter (@inbalancesa)

CHAPTER 2

ALEXANDRA ALLRED

Please tell us about your company here:

Main Street Gym is a privately owned gym outside Dallas, Texas (Midlothian). To date, I also have a Patent Pending on the PK Total Fitness system.

1. What is the best way to lose fat?

There is no single "best way." If you learn nothing else, know that your body is a machine – a wondrously complicated machine with multiple functions and pieces. To identify one sole way to efficiently burn fat is misleading and unfair to those desperate to lose weight. Just as you would work with a team to build a house, a car, or a machine, losing weight must also be a team effort and by "team" I mean combining proper diet and exercise! So ... get that in your head right now. There is no magic pill, no fast-track single exercise at the gym, etc. You have to aggressively attack from all angles to win this battle, but you can!

So how?

1. Stop justifying ... 'well, I just ran three miles, so I can eat this,' or 'one soda a day doesn't make that big of a difference."

2. Go natural. Try to find ingredients that are as close to Mother Nature as possible. Here's a clue. If you can't pronounce, much less understand what the actual ingredient is, why put it in your beautiful machine? As amazing as the United States

is, there is a reason why we are one of the unhealthiest nations in the world. For all our advances, we have become willing participants in eating whatever is handed to us. We've bought into the 'cheaper is better' motto and we're paying the price at an all-time high with medical issues that were virtually non-existent four decades ago. The average American woman is 5'4" at 140-150 pounds and a waist size of 34-35 inches. Yet four decades ago, the weight was averaged at 120 pounds with a waist size of 24-25 inches. And forty years ago, aggressive exercise and excessive sweating for a female was heavily discouraged while today we're proud of our boot camp style workouts. So, what's changed? Diet!

3. Be honest/Be Different. If gym owners, instructors, trainers around the nation were all polled and asked what is the one mistake people consistently make at the gym it would be work ethic. We have our warriors, certainly. But the majority of people are NOT working out as hard as they believe they are. Subconsciously, people feel that by simply walking through the doors of the gym or hitting the trails at the park that they are burning calories like crazy. Common complaints are always, "I come to every class, I work so hard ... why can't I lose weight?" The harsh reality is they are often working at 60 or 70% capacity. When an exercise takes a person out of his or her comfort zone, most drop off. I've had gym members faithfully attend class after class, day after day, but when they never leave the comfort zone – they don't want to let their heart rate climb too high or sweat too much or try too hard, how can they grow? [*This said – it is IMPORTANT that you have your physicians clearance if you have any medical issues and should always inform your doctor about what you are or intend to do in the way of exercise and diet.] Be honest with yourself. How hard are you working? Really?

Be different. By this, I mean ... change things up. I have a great example. I had a client who was a mail carrier. She walked a ten-mile route, five days a week and carried an (on average) 50-pound bag. When she first got the job, she lost a lot of weight and had never been so fit but over time, the weight started to come back on. By the time I met her, she was embarrassed and ashamed. "How can I be this heavy? I walk 50 miles a week!!" She was embarrassed to tell people this because when she did people would look at her critically. "How can you walk 10 miles a day and be overweight?" When I asked her what else she does in the way of workouts, she looked at me like I was crazy. I WALK TEN MILES A DAY, LADY!

Well, okay, yes, but ... she had had that route for several years. The human body is a wondrously complicated but also an adaptable machine. After several years of walking ten miles with 50 miles, it acclimated to this very quickly and up came the weight. There was no longer shock or muscle confusion to the body and less effort was required and, thus, fewer calories burned. Day in and day out, we watch as people come in and get on the same pieces of equipment, take the same classes, do the same routines and guess what? They are SO acclimated to the routine that even though they are sweating, the body is no longer struggling as it once did. You have to mix things up, create muscle confusion and a new intensity that will burn calories!

2. I have an event coming up in 2 months. What's my best strategy for getting in better shape by then?

When I hear this question, I always fire one right back: How badly do you want it? It's an important question because the answer is ... you can do incredible things in 60 days. You can do life altering, life changing things in 60 days. I watched a 280-pound woman come in every day at lunchtime and walk the treadmill at a pace so challenging that we (the staff at Main Street Gym) continuously monitored her. In less than 90 days, she lost almost 120 pounds! While this is not typical, it was inspiring and humbling to watch her want it so badly and succeed! On the flip side, while I lived in the Olympic Training Center in Lake Placid, New York, I was stunned to see elite athletes literally give up their position with a U.S. team through laziness. They took the attitude that they had it all locked up and stopped trying. Never stop trying. As the summer months wound down and new hopefuls came in, the "seasoned" athletes who hadn't been working as they should have been lost their positions to newbies who physically changed before coaches eyes in a short amount of time. It always came down to "how badly do you want it?"

If you want that gold, the best strategy is a DIFFERENT strategy. Whatever you've been doing isn't working so it's time to change things up – from how you eat to how you train. I'm not a big fan of diets or one-size-fits-all nutritional plans as they do not factor in medical issues, sleep patterns, pregnancy, nursing, age, metabolism, thyroid, etc. I do recommend finding a licensed nutritionist for a custom fit plan to you and your lifestyle. This ensures the most success. This said you can assess your own lifestyle. Are you a soda drinker? By the by, diet is WORSE. Stop it. Do you constantly load on breads and pastas? Do you skip breakfast? These are all no-nos. Eating four meals a day, as natural as possible, skipping the sodas (diet or otherwise) is the first step to igniting that metabolism. You must have fuel to burn calories and, yes, the kind of fuel you have makes a big difference. Stop telling yourself that you can eat that 250 calorie slice of pizza because you're going to burn off 300 calories later in the day. Your but-I-really-want-that logic doesn't translate the same to your machine of a body. It will store fats differently according to good and bad fats. If you want to be an efficient and lean machine, you have to give it the proper fuel. Stop telling yourself that your diet whatever doesn't have any calories. It is poison and your body – purest as it is – doesn't know what to do with the poison and shunts much of the toxic ingredients in your liver, the purifier of your system. Why, oh, why, oh, why would you do this to yourself? And so the question remains ... how much do you want this?

The second issue is the training. By putting yourself on a weight bearing, high-intensity training regiment, you will burn calories and build muscle (another fat-burning tool) to build a leaner, stronger you.

3. Is walking or running better for fat loss?

Trick question. Oh, for a penny each time a person has told they walk x-amount of miles and "nothing is happening." Then, by happenstance I see them walking and realize, 'Ahh, they are strolling!' On average when you run (jog) a mile, it is calculated (again – on average) to be 100 calories burned per mile. When you run/jog, the entire body is in play. Arms pumping, fists typically drawn up to heart level with each pump, your heart rate accelerates, muscles in the arbs, shoulders, back, and abs are working in addition to the legs. To that, the legs are working harder than normal as your foot rotation is faster. As your feet strike the surface as a faster rate, you are tapping into more muscles whereas walking – a comfortable pace – offers little more resistance than your day-to-day walking.

However, walking with purpose, the speed walker, the efficient exercising walker, is a totally different story. This walk mimics the jogger with very similar results and less pounding to the body. Those with bad ankles, knees, hips, and/or back are better suited for the walk but when they pump the arms and strive for a faster foot rotation, the walking game changes.

In the end, the jogger does more work and does burn more calories but HOW you walk determines how big the difference between jogger and walker. I taught a walking class in college – yes, there is actually such a thing – and had many students pump one pound hand weights added to the walk. When the semester began, we merely discussed stride, shoes, safety, and the pumping of arms combined with time. The object was to decrease the amount of time it took to walk a mile course. Midway into the semester, we added the one pound hand weight and oh, what a difference. Or, shall I say, oh, how people moaned and groaned. And sweated!

4. Should I do cardio or weight training?

Answer: YES! There is no either/or here. There is no sport, no elite athlete, and no dedicated competitor who focuses on sports specific skills only and neglects the weight training. He or she does not exist. From the large and powerful football player to the nymph-ish figure skater, weight training is critical to success in the sport. Weight training helps reduce risks of injury (when done properly!); it keeps muscles strong and pliable so that the athlete can perform tasks efficiently and safely with power, speed, and agility. Weight training helps balance and is an excellent tool for corrective training, that is, to help rehabilitate an injured or failing body part.

Ah, but you think that weight lifting will make you bigger and you only have two months to lose the weight you want to lose.

Remember that ice skater? Her entire career hinges on being light and agile and yet she is 100% dedicated to a regimented weight lifting routine.

When you combine weight training WITH cardio, you become that lean, fat-burning, smokin' hot machine you want to be. Assuming you have no plans to routinely powerlift your refrigerator, weight lifting creates sleek arms, toned and shapely legs, a powerful but V-shaped back with sexy shoulders and a trim waist. Truly. This is what weight lifting, complimented with cardio, is designed to do so don't be afraid to hit the weights.

For women more than men, there are two main reasons women do not lift. The first is the myth – lifting will make me bigger. False. But even when women see trim, sleek females lifting weights they are still hesitant to lift. Why? They don't know how. This is super common. In general, men gravitate to the weights and women to the classes. For women, just start slowly. Find someone who can show you what to do. In a gym, that person is most often the trainer. At home, check out some videos where 3, 5, and 10-pound weights are used. Do not be afraid to go big because it's only going to make you smaller!

On the flip side – men! What are you waiting for? While you've become accustomed to the treadmill, rowing machine, or Elliptical, it is time for you to break out of that rut and join a few classes. You will be stunned by the amount of calories you burn in class sessions. Let's face it .... You're a man. When you work out alone, there are days when you're not "feeling it," and drop off. Often times, you don't even realize how much you've dropped off. But in the class setting, you always bring your A game and boy, does that show after a few short weeks. (By the way, this is extremely irritating to the women in the classes so you might want to keep your successful and radical weight loss to yourself!)

Recently, I had a marathon runner complain to me about knee issues but was insistent that "it's not the knees but it's the knees," he'd said. He was frustrated because he did not how else to explain what he was feeling. He'd be well into the race when his quads/legs felt very heavy and a pounding feeling would develop, making each step feel burdensome. I told him he had underdeveloped hip flexors. Without getting into too much detail, the point is this: For all his running, he needed to add weight training to his routine so that when larger muscles were failing from fatigue, other primary and secondary muscles could assist. Essentially, he had no backup. By adding weight bearing hip flexor (and other) exercises to his running routine, he did, in fact, become a fast and more efficient runner. And, oh, by the way, the knee pain went away.

Again, there is no either/or here. If you want maximum results for your training efforts, combine cardio with weight training and just watch the results!!

5. What are your recommended workouts for fast results?

Muscle confusion.

Say what?

Earlier, I mentioned the 280-pound woman who dropped weight rapidly with just walking on a treadmill. It is important to note, however, that she had been completely sedentary. Just walking a quarter of a mile had been a tremendous shock to her system. Muscle confusion. Now that she has become an active person, she has begun to change up her routines. So, let's assume that we're now talking about a fairly active person who wants to drop 20 to 50 pounds. Let's play a little more and say we're talking about someone who is very active, a regular gym rat or outdoor enthusiast who wants to lose 20 pounds quickly. The answer is the same – muscle confusion. Whatever it was you were doing before has become routine and your body is acclimated to the challenges of your exercise.

You have to change things up completely. Abandon the once beloved treadmill and try out the rowing machine, skip the morning run and try out a much longer bicycle route.

I have a friend who was, by all accounts, in great shape. She was maybe five pounds overweight and very active in the gym when she decided she wanted to become a fitness model/ competitor. She was a runner. She could tackle a six-mile run and look like a newborn gazelle springing across the savannah. Less than three months later, she was a chiseled goddess and it did not come from running. In fact, from the moment she got serious about her training, she dropped all junk food and soda from her diet and ramped up her metabolism by eating six meals a day. She introduced brown rice, quinoa, and sweet potatoes as her carbohydrates and tossed the breads and pastas. She ate grilled chicken, fish, and steak and said bye-bye to the cereals, cookies, and anything processed. She cooked and grilled daily. For her exercise, the runs were out and stair climbing was in. As was, no surprise, serious weight training. She not only lost all the excess weight but developed abdominal muscles she said she never imagined she had after two children.

When asked how to get fast results, I always ask, "How badly do you want it?" For fast results, another way to ramp up the metabolism is two-a-days.

TWO-A-DAYS

Before explaining what two-a-days are, let's talk safety. Usually, I have the person who wants it buuuuut ... not really. They talk about it, think about it, ask about it but when it comes to really knuckling down and changing food habits, sleep habits, and exercise, many good intentions fade away. People don't like leaving their comfort zones, they don't like changing habits, and they don't want to work too hard for something like weight which came on with pleasant (food) memories and just hanging around. Every now and then, however, I get the super-duper enthusiastic person. I love the heart. I love to dedication. But I also worry when a person is pushing too hard. Remember that you've got to listen to and respect your body.

When you begin to feel more fatigue than normal and/or when you appear to be developing injuries, these are red flags that you are overtraining. RESPECT THE MACHINE! Hard workouts temporarily break down the body to encourage new muscle growth but this means there has to be proper recovery time so proper rest and listening to your body is vital in successful weight loss, training, and transformation experiences.

Two-a-days are just what they imply. Twice a week, serious athletes will pull a double workout in one day. This greatly ramps up the cardio, the metabolism and boosts the body to a new level. This should not be done more than twice a week if you are working out six times a week. Six times a week with two of those days being two-a-days is eight workouts in one week. Mixing weight training with varying cardio workouts is a tremendous way to ensure weight loss and/or toning.

6. How can I speed up my recovery period?

This question makes me nervous because the person asking is my Type A personality, the person who I sometimes have to kick out of my gym! While we have many who do not like to step out of their comfort zone, we also have the Type A exerciser, that person who pushes and pushes and pushes. True, this is the elite athlete mentality but if unchecked, this person can also be a danger to him or herself. Recovery is vital.

There are certainly tricks to help ensure that the body is able to recover. Sleep is NUMBER 1! Americans do not get enough sleep. Too many people have electronics in their rooms with them creating what experts call interrupted sleep. Little pings of notifications, buzzing noises and the light from electronics interrupt true sleep. Remove these things from your room. Seriously. Are you a brain surgeon? Does the future of the world rest in your hands? Are you expecting life and death phone calls or text messages? In other words, you really don't need to know what so-and-so said at midnight. It can wait until morning.

Stay hydrated. Most people have no idea how dehydrated they actually are. Check out your urine. I know, I know ... but when you use the bathroom, notice the color of your urine. If it is clear or very light yellow – fantastic. But the darker the yellow, the more dehydrated and more in distress your body is. H2O up.

Sports Drinks vs. Chocolate Milk

One of the greatest marketing ploys in the U.S. today is that of the sports drink. We've convinced ourselves that with a little sweat comes the tremendous need for a sports drink to recover. Short of you running a marathon through the desert, you don't need anything more than water. But we're guzzling sports drinks after soccer games, tennis matches, 10k races, and regular workouts in the gym because we – gasp – sweat. While attending a seminar about sports nutrition, a group of trainers and physicians got into the discussion of chocolate milk. In attendance were some of the top researchers in the field of sports medicine and nutrition and we were talking about the wonders of good old fashioned chocolate milk. While chemicals are laced in the "recovery" drinks, chocolate milk may be one of the purest, yummy recovery drinks out there. Who knew? Sometimes the most simplistic things are the very best.

Lastly, relax. Stop stressing about that timeline you've given yourself or that impending date. Do you know that you can actually slow down the weight loss process by worrying?

Your Support Group

One of the hardest things to focus on while going through any transformation is keeping things in perspective. All you focus on is the calendar and forget to give yourself credit for all the hard work and effort you are putting in. It's easy to stress out, become negative, and impede your recovery process. This is where your own support group is so necessary. This is why I am a big fan of the classroom exercise settings. Fellow gym members always notice weight loss, sliming bodies, and increased energy! If you are not a gym member, find walking or jogging buddies or some kind of support group that will take you away from the "let's do lunch," mindset and praise you for your successes – while exercising right alongside you. These little tricks will boost your energy and speed your recovery!

7. How often should I work out?

There is no hard fast rule about how often, when, and how to work out. Perhaps this is one of the reasons people struggle so much with the concept of exercise and overall fitness health. Wouldn't it be nice if there was an actual number? You must work out four times a week for 45 minutes at 80% capacity for three months before .... Blah, blah. The reality is this. All bodies are different, as are schedules, personalities, and needs. One person might truly desire to be ripped while another just wants to be able to walk around the block without gasping for breath. Every day I train college students, senior citizens, special needs young adults, at-home moms and

CEOs. Everyone wants something different. But there is one thing you can ask yourself over and over again: How much do I want this? That is the answer to the question, "How much should I work out?" If you are looking for rapid weight loss with a toned body, working out six times a week and (if you can handle it) two two-a-days is a great but hard way to shock your body into change. Please remember, however, to listen to and respect your body. Mix up the workouts, make each one challenging. If you are performing exercises but quietly thinking about what you're going to have for lunch, you may not be working as hard as you should be. Or, certainly, could be. If your "lifting weights" at the gym while reading a magazine or thumbing through your play list ... I hate to break this to ya but you're really not giving full effort there, cowboy. Make every workouts you elite-athlete workout. Believe how strong you are and test yourself. Push yourself beyond what you thought you could do. Be proud of what you can accomplish and expect nothing less. THAT is how and how often you should work out.

8. How do I get a flat stomach?

Quit the bread and run! NEXT!

(Seriously, you could do 1,000 crunches a day but if you're not changing anything else, the flat stomach is not going to happen.)

9. How do I get rid of flabby arms?

I love the arms! This is an area women are always worried about and it can be worked on quite easily.

But it is a feel first, see second deal. Whether you belong to a gym or have some hand weights at home, this is an easy area to target. If ... if ... if you are willing to make changes to the way you have been eating and are willing to work with hand weights and perform pushups, you can see a nice, very flattering improvement in the arms in 60 days. I gave the if-if-if because even if you turn into an iron-pumping, push-up performing maniac, being overweight still layers muscle. Therefore, you will FEEL the difference in your arms fairly quickly. You will feel your shoulders and triceps (back of the arm), biceps and back getting stronger and it really is empowering. But it is the fuel that you feed the machine that will help sculpt the arms the way you want them to look. Combining cardio with weight training, you can perform bicep curls, tricep kickbacks and dips, lateral raises, punches and push-ups in a series of three sets with anywhere from 12 to 20 repetitions. Do this three times a week and mark down your improvements. Keep an active journal of your workouts and mark how you grow as you move along in the next 60 days.

10. What short workouts can I do between work?

Great question. There is a variety of options. More and more companies are encouraging employees to use lunch breaks for a midday workout. If you've not heard about this at your work ... go ask. I cannot tell you how many times a member later told us that by simply approaching an employer about the idea of group exercise a new policy was put into motion. Employers are seeing (and feeling) the benefits of having healthier employees, who are also happier, have more energy, come to work with a better attitude AND insurance companies are all too happy to pay for gym memberships as they also see the monetary benefit of having healthier members. So ... ASK! This said, talk to co-workers about starting an exercise group together. As timid or embarrassed as you may feel about this, a group will ensure greater success. When you have co-workers working out with you, fewer snacks and lavish lunches will appear at work. Suddenly, the workplace will become a place of great camaraderie as you all share miles walked, lunges taken, calories burned, etc. FitBitters beware! Spontaneous competition may break out among desk mates! Bosses love this and employees need this.

Still, this may not be an option. So dig down deep and find your own motivation. Before you even begin, take a serious (and honest) look at your typical day at work. Did you go through a drive-thru on the way to work? What did you eat? Did you park right next to the office? Do you sit at your desk all day drinking diet sodas and sneaking in texts when you can? Welcome to today's corporate America. So, change things up. Demand better of yourself. Begin to knock out new challenges. Everyone wants to be told "do 15 burpees, 20 lunge steps, and 25 jumping jacks every day for 15 minutes and you will be transformed." Or "have a flat stomach in two weeks." Gee. Why didn't Oprah Winfrey with all her millions and personal trainers and private nutritionists think of that ..... The hard truth is, your hard work will pay off slowly, but it will pay off. Tell yourself you're in this for the long haul. Begin taking the stairs, park further away, no more sodas -- diet or otherwise and no more drive-thrus. With this, add mini-workouts in your day.

But first, let's get real. One of the most common "reasons" I hear for not working out is this:

"I can't work out at the gym because I'm at work all day ... but I can't get sweaty at work."

My answer:

If you really want it, you will find a way. Olympic athlete moms who also work full-time jobs find a way to work out at 4 am or 10 pm. They find a way to slip in workouts at or around work.

They are super busy. They get sweaty. But they want it. Want it. Want it badly enough that you are willing to inconvenience that schedule that has clearly not been working for you up to this point. Shuffle the deck. Change the rules. You CAN do this.

There is no ONE single way to work out in the middle of the day. You can run stairs, walk, do lunges. You can do a pyramid workout for 15 minutes:

20 seconds of sit ups

20 seconds of push ups

20 seconds of lunges

20 seconds of burpees or jumping jacks

40 seconds of sit ups

40 seconds of push ups

40 seconds of lunges

40 seconds of burpees or jumping jacks

1 minute of sit ups

1 minute of push-ups (even if you can only knock out four in 60 seconds, count that and try to improve next time!)

1-minute lunges

1 minute of burpees or jacks

40 seconds of sit ups

40 seconds of push ups

40 seconds of lunges

40 seconds of burpees or jumping jacks

20 seconds of sit ups

20 seconds of push ups

20 seconds of lunges

20 seconds of burpees or jumping jacks = 12 minutes/approx 15 with transitions!

Whatever it is your do .... commit. Want it. Believe that you can and just do it!

11. What is the best diet to follow?

I HATE this questions ... okay, not really. I'm glad you asked, but it is so complicated. Every body is different. Every need is different. For some, the need is to tone rather than lose. Others may need only to lose a few pounds while others are looking at over 50 pounds and how (and what) you eat relates to your energy levels. How you work out dictates how you should be eating. Too many "dieters" come to the gym and tap out in about 22 minutes with so little energy, they cannot even see how inefficient their exercise actually is. They were better off taking a nap than coming to the gym.

Dieting isn't the answer. A lifestyle change is the answer and here's why. Okay, so you really only want to make a big change for the next 60 days, right? Wrong. The reality is, you want to get into shape (whatever that ideal is for you) within the next 60 days for that very important date. But you still have a problem; you are or were still at a point that you need some emergency "fix." This would indicate that should you return to the way you were living, eating, sleeping, working, training will lead you right back to where you were.

This is where the term yo-yo dieting comes from. You get serious for two months and then go right back to old [bad] habits.

Instead, think of a lifestyle change. Write down the things that you consume, drink, and food that you know to be unhealthy, unwise, harmful, inefficient fuel. Keep that list on your fridge, share with family members, and discuss how you all can slowly eliminate these things from your diet.

Take a hard look at how you get your food. Are you cooking or picking up fast food? Buying prepackaged/processed meals or using fresh ingredients?

As you eliminate more and more unhealthy foods, your taste will change. Suddenly, you will start to crave things you've never craved before. As your body adjusts to healthy, real foods, it will want the better product! It then becomes cyclical. You will continue to burn fuel (and fat) more efficiently, you'll retain less water, your body will begin to shed pounds, and even your skin texture will change. It is a beautiful thing to watch a person become healthy – really healthy. And as easy as it's been stated here, it truly begins by simply eliminating bad things from your diet and adding in healthy, natural foods.

12. Do I need to take dietary supplements?

Another trick question. If you are eating well, getting balanced meals and are well hydrated, the going theory is that you will be consuming enough proper nutrients. But ... you may have medical issues that require something extra. Almost 40% of American women are anemic and many have no idea. They just think they're tired from lack of sleep. As you begin this journey, make an appointment with your primary physician to have a wellness check-up. Use this time to discuss any medical issues you may have and suggested supplements, if needed.

THIS SAID ... let's have a little talk about supplements to "help you lose weight." I cannot even begin to describe my distain for these products. At the store, rows and rows of boxes proclaim, "Lose weight while you sleep," "Drop ten pounds instantly," or my personal favorite, "Lose weight without working out!" Forget the fact that you're putting chemicals into your body, that many such products also come with disclaimers about what ingesting this little miracle pill can do to your heart, head, vision, organs, even causing dizziness or diarrhea. ARE YOU SERIOUS? Never mind all these terrifying prospects that you are so willing to do to your one and only body rather than just put in hard, honest work. The absolute best argument I have against these little spawns of Satan is this ... years ago Oprah Winfrey, named the wealthiest woman in the United States stated that with her very well documented battle with weight and all her resources and money, if there were a miracle pill out there she would buy the company. But no such pill exists.

13. What tips do you have for healthy food on the go?

We all get lazy. It is much easier to buy something while you're out, but the truth is, nothing beats preparing meals ahead of time and taking them with you. This said we all have that time when we just could not or did not prepare something and we're starved. So, what do you eat? The safest answer is to select things that are as close to nature as possible. Nuts, salads, fruits, and vegetables are always safe and today's markets and even gas stations carry such things.

Many times, however, you'll find yourself in a fast food restaurant with children. Understandable. So, again, what do you get? The grilled chicken seems safe, right? Not so fast. Ever wonder how those chicken breasts, sitting under the heating lamps stay so juicy? Most chicken breasts are injected with beef broth to keep the flavor. If the food is in a fast food establishment, it is a fairly safe bet that it is not entirely natural. Stick to what you know. Salad. Veggies. Do NOT look at this as a punishment but, rather, having dodged a disgusting bullet. When you make the full commitment to healthy eating, it empowers you when you can turn something away. And I have never heard a lead in for the 10 o'clock news that read: A woman chose not to eat a grilled chicken patty and died right there on the spot.

14. Who is your ideal client to work with?

I tell my classes all the time ... "I can teach your proper form and technique. I can explain how to use equipment and what muscles you are working. I can teach you all these things, but I can't teach you heart. That's all you." My ideal student is someone who is invested in the idea of the journey and not the magic pill. There is an interesting difference between my senior citizens and college students. While the college student is young, healthy, and (in theory) strong, today's youth is full of excuses. "I couldn't come because ..." "I didn't do that because ..." while my seniors, with limited physical abilities, vision, with cancer or artificial body parts are always on time, always present, always smiling and eager to work. I am so less interested in how much you can bench press but so much more invested in your attitude!

15. What are the main benefits of working with a personal trainer?

A trainer can keep your routines fresh and fun while challenging your body. A trainer can keep you honest, correcting and perfecting your form while also motivating you to stay to a schedule. But a trainer can also tell when you lagging from exhaustion, from a poor diet, from injury or laziness. These are important distinctions because there will be times when you would swear you were working as hard as you ever have but, in truth, your energy stores are so low that you're not doing nearly the work you think you are. These are the times when a conversation with a professional can be what it takes to lose weight in the following week or break through to a new threshold. If no one is there to challenge you and question your form and energy, it is much harder to grow. This said you do not have to have a trainer. It helps but if you have that heart, that motivation, that go-for-the-gold attitude, you can succeed alone!

Please tell us how readers can get in contact with you here:

I can always be contacted through the Main Street Gym website at www.mainstgym.net or my own website at www. alexandratheauthor.com

CHAPTER 3

BRIAN STERLING-VETE

Please tell us about your company here:

MajorVision has been trading successfully since 1992 and provides a select range of personal coaching services to clients on an international basis.

1. What is the best way to lose fat?

The best way to lose fat is to simply reduce your calorie intake below the point where you eat just enough to maintain your bodyweight, while at the same time increase your Base Metabolic Rate (BMR) through exercise.

When looking at your Base Metabolic Rate or BMR, one first has to understand what your Metabolism actually is; which is basically the chemical reactions taking place in your cells which provide the energy to sustain and maintain your life. Therefore, in simple terms your BMR is the rate at which your body burns energy to carry out the functions related to maintaining your life. For the average person this means that about 20% of energy is burned during daily activities, and obviously this percentage rises according to the amount and intensity of the exercises performed during your workout sessions. Assuming that you use 10% of energy to digest and process the food you eat, the remaining percentage of energy which for a person who doesn't exercise would be 70%, would be then burned during your rest periods of the day. This is your BMR and the faster your BMR burns energy, the more efficiently your body burns energy. The more muscle mass you have, the faster your BMR will be. Therefore, a major benefit of exercising to add muscle is the natural side-effect of burning more energy as a result which equals fat loss. As a person ages, they often lose lean muscle mass, so their BMR slows as part of the process which is just one of the reasons why it's very important to exercise regularly throughout your life. Your body has certain auto response defense mechanisms, one of which slows your BMR rapidly if you crash diet and eat virtually nothing. Your body's mechanism which has developed over thousands of years of evolution believes there's a famine and automatically conserves your energy reserves to preserve your life until the famine is over. In short, crash diets don't work very well.

Certain exercises are better than others and people often have misconceptions about exercises such as sit-ups/trunk curls. The fact is that sit-ups/trunk curls burn fewer calories and provide less stimulus for your BMR than exercises such as squats, deadlift, chin ups and bench press. The more lean muscle that you have, the greater your Base Metabolic rate will be, therefore just by being more muscular, you'll burn more calories while at rest. Use short Burst Training/High-Intensity Interval training routines which have a greater long-term post-exercise fat burning effect than the traditional aerobic exercise model.

Short Burst Training or SBT and High-Intensity Interval training are essentially the same thing. The principle is a variant of circuit training which includes a series of high-intensity bursts of exercise movements of short durations of time interwoven into a lower intensity exercise session. Depending upon the intensity of the exercise and the equipment used, the short bursts of high-intensity exercise would usually last for between 30 and 60 seconds. The process is repeated several times during a workout session, with the overall length of workout and the number of short bursts sessions included in each workout being directly dependent upon the intensity of the bursts themselves. People might more commonly refer to a High-intensity Interval Training workout or HIIT workout when an exercise session starts with a warm-up period of some sort leading into a single high-intensity exercise period, which then leads into a cool-down period to conclude the workout. Once again, the high-intensity exercise are performed at near maximum capacity, which is directly reflected in the duration of the period itself.

2. I have an event coming up in 2 months. What's my best strategy for getting in better shape by then?

Planning is everything if you have a specific target in mind. However, before any effective plan can be drawn up, an honest and accurate assessment of one's current status must be determined. For example, it's no use 'believing' that you're in 'pretty good shape' when in reality you're in terrible shape. Once you've determined your current, accurate physical condition, then draw up a REALISTIC plan to achieve a REALISTIC shape in 2 months' time. If weight loss is your goal, then don't expect to lose more than between 1 and 2 lbs per week depending upon your diet and exercise routine. Remember that since you have to burn 3,500 calories to burn just one pound of fat, then to lose 1.5lbs would mean burning 5000 calories more than you ingest. With your realistic diet plan in place, next draw up a realistic exercise routine. If you goal is to look more muscular, then took a high-intensity weight training routine. Alternatively, if your goal is just to look, fitter, then look towards a Burst Training/High-intensity Interval training routine.

3. Is walking or running better for fat loss?

Both walking and running are an excellent way to burn calories, tone up and promote weight loss, however, there are distinct benefits to each. In simple terms running burns more calories than walking does, however walking burns more fat than running because when exercising at a lower intensity fat is actually being used as the fuel. When you shift gears and increase from walking to running, then your body burns more carbohydrates as fuel. In overall terms it doesn't matter much if you're burning fat or using carbohydrate as the primary fuel; what is important, however, is that you burn the most calories during your exercise session. Therefore, even though walking may burn more fat as fuel, running will burn more overall calories. Another important factor to consider when looking at the differences between walking and running are the risks of injury from each. Overall, in simple terms running carries more risk of injury than walking does.

4. Should I do cardio or weight training?

In simple terms, cardiovascular training burns more calories than weight training. However for serious calorie burning High-intensity Interval Training will ensure that more overall calories are burned during the combined exercise and 24-hour post exercise period than by performing just regular cardiovascular exercises.

5. What are your recommended workouts for fast results?

The best overall workouts for getting fast result are Short Burst Training and High-intensity Training, with the latter referring to purely weight training. The best regimen would include High-intensity Interval Training to maximise the calories burned together with a high-intensity weight training routine to stimulate the maximum possible muscular gains. Keep your workouts short, focussed and intense.

6. How can I speed up my recovery period?

After high-intensity training, muscles can require anything from 24 to 48 hours recovery time in order to repair and rebuild tissue. Working out too frequently will simply deplete muscle tissue and have the opposite effect to what you wish to achieve. To speed up recovery time make sure that you're properly hydrated because water supports nutrient transfer in the body which is essential when speeding up your recovery time.

Eat high quality food within an hour of ending your exercise session. This is very important because it helps your body to repair and recover faster which means that you'll receive faster results and greater benefits from your hard workout sessions. After exercise, you want your food to be absorbed as rapidly as possible to begin the repair and recovery processes right away, so the type of food you choose is obviously very important. You certainly want to avoid refined carbohydrates and sugars which will raise your blood sugars levels too rapidly and, therefore, increase the chances of storing more body fat. Since your body will need a complete range of essential amino acids as well as other vitamins and nutrients, I recommend a water-based shake such as Garden of Life's Raw Meal and Raw Protein, of a mix of the two. These products have the added benefits of being both organic and vegan, with the latter negating the negative impact which dairy has on the body. The 30 to 60-minute window for eating post-exercise reflects the results of certain studies which indicate when the body begins to draw upon itself to repair and recover from the exercise session. If the body doesn't receive the nutrients it needs from an external source, then the benefits gained from your hard workout sessions are reduced.

Incorporate a proper stretching routine after your workout session. Get plenty of quality sleep and rest time. While you sleep, your body produces Growth Hormone, which will repair and build tissue.

7. How often should I workout?

This all depends on how intense your workouts are. In simple terms the higher the intensity of the workout, then the shorter the workout will be and the longer the rest time needed in order for the body to recover, repair and rebuild before another workout can be performed. A realistic assessment has to be made of the each individual's current condition and also about what they consider to be a high-intensity workout. Once this has been determined, then a plan can be drawn up to schedule regular workouts. For most people, performing a full body workout session each time, this will mean they work out between two and four times per week depending upon the intensity of each session. For most people in practical terms, a full body workout of reasonable intensity can be performed 3 times per week with one day of rest between each session and two days over the weekend.

8. How do I get a flat stomach?

To achieve a flat stomach means a combination of healthy low-calorie eating, burning body fat, increasing your Base Metabolic Rate and performing the right exercises. Avoid over-eating which will stretch the stomach, and avoid drinking too much fluid as this will stretch the stomach and contribute to the classic 'beer-belly' effect. Keep in mind that you're dealing with a combination of excess Visceral fat which surrounds the organs, excess Subcutaneous Fat which is between the skin and muscles and basically forms the outer wrapping of the muscles under the skin, and Intramuscular Fat which is the fat within the muscle itself and has the visual appearance of marbling.

9. How do I get rid of flabby arms?

To eliminate flabby arms requires all of the above in section 8. Flabby arms are simply the result of excess subcutaneous fat and also intramuscular fat. Reducing both kinds of fat will firm up flabby arms and to reduce the fat it requires burning calories and exercise.

10. What short workouts can I do between work?

The best short workouts to do between work are bodyweight and self-resistance workouts. A bodyweight workout is one that doesn't require weights or equipment and relies on an individual's own body weight as resistance. Self-resistance training (SRT) is the practice of purely using one's own self to produce the necessary resistance. This means pitting muscle against opposing muscle. Both forms of exercise are effective and can be done between work. Certain new simple, yet highly effective devices which help both forms of exercise have been released on to the market in recent years. The most highly recommended are the Iso-Gym which is a self-resistance and bodyweight exercise device which is extremely compact and highly effective. The other is the Iso-Bow, which literally easily fits into your pocket and yet can make self-resistance exercises so effective that they can be performed with equal efficiency by Olympic athletes or by a senior citizen.

11. What is the best diet to follow?

The best diet to follow is the one which you'll stick to and maintain. If you attempt a diet which you won't stick to, then it's simply a waste of time and effort.

A good diet follows the principles of:

- Excellent nutrition

- Low calorie

- High fibre

- Low fat

- Protein rich

- Free from processing and additives

- An excellent balance of fruits, raw vegetables, and minimal meat – preferably only seafood

12. Do I need to take dietary supplements?

People take dietary supplements to ensure they get enough essential nutrients to maintain or improve their health. However, not everyone needs to take supplements and there can even be a risk of negative side-effects to some supplements in certain individuals. In theory it's possible to get all of the nutrients you need by eating a variety of healthy foods, so you don't have to take any supplements, however, modern food storage, and transportation and lead to gaps in our nutrition which is where supplements can help. Excessive use of protein supplements can be damaging and slow your metabolism, especially if you follow a high-protein diet for longer than a few months. Physically active adults should eat approximately 0.5 grams of protein per pound of bodyweight, while those people building muscle mass should eat up to 1 gram per pound of bodyweight. Therefore a 150-pound average physically active adult would require between 75 and 150 grams of protein per day.

13. What tips do you have for healthy food on the go?

My best tips for healthy food on the go would be Raw Meal by Garden of Life. It's an excellent, well-balanced super nutritious shake. It mixes with water easily, it's low in calories, high in rice fibre to take away the feelings of hunger and it provides a complete spectrum of amino acids while at the same time being both organic and vegan. The Raw Protein from the same company is also excellent and bot or a mix of both will provide excellent nutrition 'on the go.' As someone who travels frequently by air, it's no problem carrying a Smart Shaker (from Smart Shake) containing several portions of either in sections because they meet TSA carry-on requirements. This means that once through airport security you can simply add water from a drinking fountain and you have a full day of excellent nutrition even on a transatlantic flight. You also avoid low-quality airline food and over-priced air-side restaurants.

14. Who is your ideal client to work with?

My ideal client is one who is dedicated to doing whatever it takes to achieve the results they desire. My personal ideal client was also someone who became a good friend, Jon Pall Sigmarsson. He was the most focused, dedicated and driven individual I've ever had the privilege to work with; which is also one reason why he was the 4 x time winner of the World's Strongest Man contest.

15. What are the main benefits of working with a personal trainer?

The main benefits of working with a personal trainer are:

- Getting fast, safe and efficient results

- You don't have to be an expert in exercise and nutrition, leave that to your trainer

- You'll learn new routines and skills

- Your trainer will be better able to maintain a balanced overview of your requirements and progress

- You'll benefit from a buddy system and be more motivated as a result

- You'll skip fewer workouts than if you train alone

- You'll train harder and more intensely

Please tell us how readers can get in contact with you here:

Website: http: //www.briansterlingvete.com

Facebook: https: //www.facebook.com/pages/Brian-Sterling-Vete/683306315093619

CHAPTER 4

DR RICHARD E. HARRIS II & KEEON RUDDER

Please tell us about your company here:

1) VonElijahFitness.com help mommies lose the baby weight from the comfort of their homes

2) VEfit help brides look their absolute best on their wedding day

3) Subscribers can ask our team of doctors any kid, health, injury, or fitness question (i.e. a Chiropractor, a Pediatrician, & a General Practitioner)

1. What is the best way to lose fat?

The best way for someone to lose fat is to lower their caloric intake. Most people don't realize how many extra calories they intake above what is needed for their particular level of activity. A 5-10% reduction in caloric intake, below what a person needs per day, can lead to fat loss. This, of course, needs to be combined with a resistance training and cardio program.

2. I have an event coming up in 2 months. What's my best strategy for getting in better shape by then?

Fitness is a lifestyle choice that we desperately need. The

rates of obesity are steadily increasing which can cause a staggering increase in healthcare cost and lost productivity. It is recommended someone not put a tremendous amount of pressure on them self to meet a 2-month deadline to get in shape. The best thing one can do is find a training and diet regimen that they can stick with over the long-term and start today.

3. Is walking or running better for fat loss?

Both walking and running can be great for fat loss but make sure to incorporate variations in training intensity and intervals. If someone chooses to walk for cardio, it is recommended they walk at an incline for 30 to 45 minutes. Cardio performed for a long distance at a consistent pace destroys the body's muscles and will lead to a "skinny fat" appearance. Interval training for 20 minutes is highly effective for fat loss.

4. Should I do cardio or weight training?

Both cardio and weight training are necessary for well-rounded fitness.

5. What are your recommended workouts for fast results?

I don't tend to recommend workouts for fast results. Fitness is a lifestyle and acclimation to a new lifestyle takes a little time. Instead, I usually have people set goals for 3 months, 6 months, 9 months, and 12 months. To get the most out of your lifestyle change you have to combine an achievable nutrition, cardio, and workout regimen.

6. How can I speed up my recovery period?

To speed up your body's recovery period, stay hydrated during the day. Also, there is a lot of data that suggest the consumption of creatine after exercise can aid muscle recovery. Next, you want to eat at least 20 grams of protein and 35 grams of carbs after resistance training for optimal muscle growth.

Try to eat the lion's share of your carbs before and right after you exercise.

7. How often should I workout?

The 2008 Physical activity guidelines recommended at people to work out at least 150 minutes a week via moderate intensity exercise, which includes walking. However, contemporary guidelines recommend a person exercise at least 300 minutes a week, which is roughly 5 days a week of 60-minute sessions.

8. How do I get a flat stomach?

The holy grail of resistance training. To get a flat stomach requires strict adherence to a diet, resistance training, and cardio program. Doing long distance cardio at a steady pace can actually impair your stomach as your cortisol levels spike, which leads to deposition of fat in the abdominal area. Equally as important, make sure you train upper abs, lower abs, oblique, and the transverse ab muscles. There are so many more tips and tricks, but those are the basics.

9. How do I get rid of flabby arms?

To get rid of flabby arms, train your legs and every other body part in addition to your arms. As you build muscle mass, your body will become more efficient at burning fat, which will reduce your overall body fat composition.

10. What short workouts can I do between work?

The best short workout to do in between work is circuit training if you are crunched for time. Exercise two muscle groups each day and alternate between the two muscle groups without taking a rest or a break in between sets. Circuit training reduces your aggregate workout time and can allow you to jam-pack a lot of exercises into one day's workout. Also, cardio interval training can be ideal for someone on a time crunch.

11. Do I need to take dietary supplements?

The million dollar question – Do you need to take dietary supplements? The answer is yes, no, and maybe. Protein supplementation after working out is essential, but you can consume protein from a multitude of sources other than simply via a shake. Although protein shakes has a major advantage of fast absorption, animal proteins are always preferred over supplements. For example, you can either eat 20 g of animal protein after you workout or drink a 20 g protein shake. In addition, there is good data that states creatine can help increase muscle mass and it can help someone recover after exercising. Be aware, high-intensity exercise programs can cause oxidative stress on the body but multivitamins can aid in recovery. Fish oil has anti-inflammatory properties and there is a lot of new evidence stating that your gut bacteria can influence metabolism as well. However, are all of these supplements necessary if you adhere to your diet and exercise program? There are plenty of people who do well without supplements and there are a ton of people who do well with them.

12. What is the best diet to follow?

The best diet to follow will vary depending on the person's activity level. The person who is more active should eat more protein and carbs (especially before and after they workout). People who are less active should have higher protein diets and eat fewer carbs and those carbs should be the slow releasing carbs like brown rice and sweet potatoes for example. A person's fat intake can remain pretty constant as long as they are eating good fats.

13. What tips do you have for healthy food on the go?

It is absolutely okay to dine out every once in awhile but always check the caloric content of the

food and make sure you adjust your total calories for the rest of the day to more accurately reflect the on-the-go meal you consumed. Also, tote items like almonds, protein shakes, or protein bars which are all high in fiber and serve as excellent snacks in between meals.

14. Who is your ideal client to work with?

The ideal client is motivated, driven, and accomplishes their goals without the need of a micro manager. It is an absolute pleasure to teach a client who has the desire to achieve their goals but simply lack the know-how; clients as such are hungry for transformation and their eagerness to learn make the trainer's life much easier.

15. What are the main benefits of working with a personal trainer?

Studies have shown that people who work out with a personal trainer are more likely to workout with some degree of extrinsic motivation. Working out with a personal trainer also gives the lifter an advantage of having someone there to spot them and assess their form for discrepancies that could possibly lead to injury. Keep in mind, every sport has a learning curve but personal trainers can help someone overcome the learning curve safely and quickly.

Please tell us how readers can get in contact with you here:

Phone: (281) 756-7885

Instagram: Von_Elijah_Fitness

Facebook: facebook.com/VonElijahllc

Twitter: twitter.com/VonElijahllc

Website: VonElijahFitness.com

CHAPTER 5

ALEX PERRY

Please tell us about your company here:

Character Strength & Conditioning is a small business that uses Strength & Conditioning as a basis for Personal Development and growth. As part of the Character Strength Family you don't just get fitter and stronger, you learn about living a healthy lifestyle, building a better life for yourself, and using what you learn to help and empower others.

1. What is the best way to lose fat?

Without a doubt the best way to lose fat is to remove as much sugar as possible from your diet! That means cutting out sweets, chocolate, cakes, fizzy drinks, fruit juice and everything else that's full of sugar. Your body doesn't need it and it's stopping you losing weight.

2. I have an event coming up in 2 months. What's my best strategy for getting in better shape by then?

Your best strategy will be to combine good quality food with a good quality exercise routine. Basically you'll be trying to eat fresh, natural, healthy food whilst challenging yourself physically at least three times per week. No fad diets, no 'miracle cures', just hard work and common sense.

3. Is walking or running better for fat loss?

Technically running burns more calories, so I'll say running. However, what's most important with any exercise is that you can regularly repeat it. So if you don't like running, or you have bad knees, then stick to walking.

4. Should I do cardio or weight training?

Whilst cardio can be great, I personally recommend weight training as your main focus. With weight training, you'll be burning calories in the session as well as after the session whilst your muscles recover. You can always add in extra sessions of light cardio if you want the extra challenge each week.

5. What are your recommended workouts for fast results?

I LOVE workouts that mix up sets, reps, and intensity. I'll usually get my clients warmed up then perform 2-3 heavy sets of 4-6 squats. I'll then get them doing some circuits of three or four exercises. So for example that might mean lunges, dumbbell overhead presses, kettlebell swings and cable rows. I'll get them performing about 15 repetitions of each exercise back to back with no rest. I might then finish the session off with some sprints or burpees! The variety really forces your body to adapt and change.

6. How can I speed up my recovery period?

Three simple things make a world of difference. Firstly you'll need to make sure you get at least 8 hours sleep each night. This allows your body to properly rest, repair and rebuild itself. Secondly you'll want to make sure your nutrition is good. Fresh meats and vegetables will help you recover much better than coffee and cake! Lastly I'd recommend some gentle foam rolling and stretching, it really helps to relax your muscles and improve your blood flow.

7. How often should I workout?

This is a tough question because it's really specific to you as an individual. Personally I'd say start with twice per week and see how you feel. If you feel good after a few weeks, then try three sessions per week. Always make sure you're recovering well between your sessions, sometimes less is more.

8. How do I get a flat stomach?

Weight loss and Stomach Vacuum Exercises! (Don't worry I'll explain below) Unfortunately there's no way to specifically target the fat around your stomach, it will come off as you lose weight and nothing you can do will make that happen differently.

However, what you can do is train your Transverse Abdominus (TVA for short) which is a deeper core muscle that acts as your body's own 'weight belt' and naturally draws your stomach in. I recommend stomach vacuums as an exercise for this. Basically you'll breathe in as you expand your belly, then breathe out as you suck your belly in and hold nice and tight. I recommend five holds of 5 to 10 seconds for beginners. Have a quick look on Google for a demonstration.

9. How do I get rid of flabby arms?

As with your stomach, you can't specifically target fat in any one area so the fat on your arms will come off as you lose weight.

Again, though, what you can do is train your arm muscles to add a bit of definition to your arms. Some simple tricep and bicep exercises will help with this.

10. What short workouts can I do between work?

I'd say go for some High-intensity Circuits. High-intensity means you'll be aiming to get your heart rate above 80% of maximum. (You shouldn't be able to talk!) I recommend picking 4 of 5 tough exercises and performing them back to back with little or no rest to form 1 round. For your full workout, I'd suggest you complete 3 to 5 rounds with about 60 seconds recovery in between. This type of high-intensity training is great because it challenges your muscles as well as your heart and lungs, meaning you'll burn through calories! It's also really quick so you can fit in a great workout even if you've only got half an hour.

11. What is the best diet to follow?

The 'No-Diet' diet. Honestly the most important thing to learn about achieving and staying at a healthy weight is that DIETS DO NOT WORK IN THE LONG TERM. Most people lose loads of weight then rebound and put it all back on.

What you need is a lifestyle change that involves common sense and the 80/20 rule. Basically this means 80% of the stuff you eat should be good quality food. So 80% will be fresh vegetables, meat, eggs, nuts, seeds, pulses, and all the stuff we know are good for us. The other 20% can be whatever you want it to be.

The reason most diets fail in the long term is because they're just not sustainable. They remove too much food or they're too restrictive. The 80/20 rule works because it's sustainable long term. You'll look better, feel better, lose weight and yet still be allowed to have a slice of cake a couple of times a week!

12. Do I need to take dietary supplements?

To cut a long story short, NO. They're mainly just expensive wastes of money. A good nutrition plan full of fresh vegetables should give you everything you need.

The only thing I might recommend is Fish oil for your Omega 3's, especially if you're vegetarian or vegan.

13. What tips do you have for healthy food on the go?

Be prepared. I always advise my clients to prepare lots of healthy food in one go. So if they're making a tuna and vegetable salad, I tell them to make three times the amount and store it in the fridge. That way they can grab a healthy snack to take with them anytime they go out.

14. Who is your ideal client to work with?

When I say, I'm a Strength & Conditioning Coach people tend to assume that I only work with men or that I only work with athletes. That is completely false.

I actually work with a huge range of both men and women from the ages of 16 through 60. My ideal client is simply someone who works hard, who listens to the advice I give them and who comes to every session with a good attitude.

15. What are the main benefits of working with a personal trainer?

I could go on for days. First and foremost it means you've got someone there to teach you correct form and technique, which are the foundations of an effective workout. You've also got someone to design programmes for you and give you specific advice about the types of exercise and food that suit you as an individual.

Most importantly, though, is that you've got someone to motivate you and keep you moving towards your goals. We all have bad days and we all have times that we feel like giving up, but a good personal trainer or coach will help you overcome those feelings and push you to achieve your dreams.

Please tell us how readers can get in contact with you here:

You can contact me directly, alex@characterstrength.co.uk

or you can visit my website, www.characterstrength.co.uk

You'll also find me on YouTube.com/characterstrength and on Facebook.com/characterstrength

CHAPTER 6

BRANDON ROBERTS

Please tell us about your company here:

Brandon Roberts is a doctoral student in Muscle Biology at the University of Florida. He has worked as a personal trainer for the past 5 years and is part of the Strength and Conditioning staff at the University of Florida. He offers online personal training and works as a fitness writer.

1. What is the best way to lose fat?

The best way to lose fat is to eat at a caloric deficit. Repeated studies have shown that having excess body fat is a result of eating and storing more calories than one burn. By doing this you put your body in a state of negative energy balance, where it doesn't have energy it needs to perform normal tasks such as moving. However, your body won't just shut down in a caloric deficit. Instead it will use your stored body fat for energy and as a result you will lose weight (specifically, fat). This is why a caloric deficit is essential to losing weight.

In order not to lose muscle mass, aim for a loss of 1-2% of bodyweight per week. There is no magic diet that will help you lose weight, but rather most diets work by limiting some type of macronutrient. Eating too many calories, even from whole or organic foods, doesn't make it better for your body in terms of fat storage. It will still cause fat gain. The most common diets limit carbohydrate or fat intake since excess protein is excreted out of the body as urea. The key is to find something that won't cause you to become irritable and focus on food every minute of the day. Some people work better on certain diets, but it's up to you to figure out which one is best for your daily lifestyle.

Other than dieting, exercise can help increase your energy expenditure, consequently burning calories. Even the smallest amount of exercise can help you create a negative energy balance. As you exercise more and at higher intensity levels, you burn more calories. Also, there is no special exercise/ workout/plan that you need to do. Find what works for you.

A healthy approach is the best approach. The best way to lose fat and keep it off is to do something sustainable and to change your lifestyle to something that is both enjoyable and rewarding.

2. I have an event coming up in 2 months. What's my best strategy for getting in better shape by then?

I recommend to start exercising and tracking what you eat. Two months is a short amount of time, but it is possible to lose 10-15lbs in a healthy way. The easiest thing to do for most people is to cut out soda, alcohol, sweets and any other calorie dense snacks. Replace these with vegetables and a few pieces of fruit. Focus on eating regularly every 3-4 hours so that you don't binge eat when hungry and make smart, healthy choices.

As for exercise, I would recommend starting slowly to prevent injury or burn-out. A lot of people go full speed and end up crashing early. Remember, you want something sustainable. If new to exercise, start with some simple cardio (i.e., walking/ jogging/cycling) 2-3 days a week for 30-45 minutes and 1-2 sessions of resistance training per week. As you find yourself getting in better shape increase the intensity of your workouts.

3. Is walking or running better for fat loss?

Walking and running can both be very good for fat loss. While running burns more calories in a shorter amount of time, they both cause similar metabolic responses. If you don't currently run, start with walking to prevent injury. If you have minimal time to devote to working out then try sprints/running. Always remember to slowly progress any exercise so your body has time to adapt.

4. Should I do cardio or weight training?

You should do both. The benefits of cardiovascular training are based on the heart which is great for overall health. Furthermore, weight training provides function for everyday tasks and helps decrease the chance of general injury. A good balance will benefit overall health.

5. What are your recommended workouts for fast results?

I recommend doing strength circuits for the fastest results. These focus on compound lifting movements such as the squat and deadlift. For example, to hit all the main muscle groups I would do these three exercises with weights: squats, bench press, and row. These movements are very taxing and should be done with proper form to prevent injury. I would recommend doing 3 sets of 12 repetitions with 2-3 minute rests. The goal is to keep your heart rate elevated and using the weights for metabolic conditioning. This type of training will cause your muscles to grow stronger because of the weight, but it will also allow you to get the benefits of cardio since it is high tempo.

6. How can I speed up my recovery period?

The best way to recover is with adequate nutrition and rest. For the general population that is all you need. Some athletes benefit from ice baths and massages, but these only provide minimal recovery. It is important to sleep 7-8 hours per night and abstain from alcohol when recovering from intense activity. Proper hydration is also essential, I recommend drinking 80-100oz of water per day.

7. How often should I workout?

I recommend working out 3-5 times per week for a healthy person. It can vary tremendously but learn to understand the signals of your body. It is important to know the difference between muscle fatigue and laziness. If your joints and muscles start to become achy, it may be time for a day off. On the other hand, it is important to push yourself in the gym since that will force your body to adapt. If you've never exercised, start with 1-2 days per week. After a month increase that to 2-3 days. Then adjust accordingly for your goals.

8. How do I get a flat stomach?

The saying goes "Abs are made in the kitchen". This is completely true. To get a flat stomach, you need to lose adipose tissue around your waistline. However, there is no way to directly target stomach fat. This could be the first or last place that you lose fat. Therefore, if you exercise and have healthy eating habits to cause weight loss, your stomach will eventually be flat.

9. How do I get rid of flabby arms?

Unfortunately, there is no way to directly target areas for "spot reduction". However, if you lose fat, flabby arms will eventually disappear. The location that your body loses fat varies for each person.

Don't get discouraged if you still have flabby arms; instead take measurements with a tape ruler to see where else you may be losing the inches.

10. What short workouts can I do between work?

Any workout can be a good workout, whether that's climbing the stairs for 30 minutes or going to the gym on your lunch hour. The key is to fully complete your workout rather than skip the last few exercises because you have to get back to work. If you have an hour lunch break, then that is enough time to do resistance exercise, including a proper warm-up and cool down. If not, it might be best to use this time for cardiovascular exercise such as jogging or cycling.

11. What is the best diet to follow?

I think the best diet to follow is one that you can stick to. Whether that's a low carb diet, low-fat diet, or anything else. I am an avid believer in IIFYM (if it fits in your macros). This is the theory that you can eat whatever you want as long as it fits in your macronutrient content for the day. Macronutrients are protein, carbohydrates, and fats. Eating clean, healthy food can certainly help you lose weight and burn fat, but there is no magical connection between healthy food and weight loss. Eat the foods you love, stay within your own macronutrient range and lose weight without the pain that most people associate with dieting!

12. Do I need to take dietary supplements?

Definitely not. Supplements should fill any gaps that you might have in your diet, but are by no means necessary. There are only a few supplements that are scientifically proven to help. One of those is whey protein, which increase muscle protein synthesis. This will help your muscles recover from the workout by giving it building blocks to repair itself. Another supplement that can enhance over-all workload during resistance training is creatine monohydrate. Caffeine, in moderation, can block drowsiness and help with overall energy levels throughout the day and during exercise. These are non-essential and I would recommend focusing on your general diet rather than supplements to achieve any fitness goals.

13. What tips do you have for healthy food on the go?

Meal prep! It's the number one thing to plan for when on the go. I find it easiest to plan my day by incorporating meal-time into the routine. It's just so important to eat right, wherever you may be. If eating out, you want to know the content of what you're eating. A lot of restaurants have nutrition facts on their websites or even on the menus. Be aware of what you're eating, just because a salad is "healthy" doesn't mean that it has a good calorie content.

14. Who is your ideal client to work with?

I don't have an ideal client. I am willing to work with anyone that is dedicated to bettering themselves. I like having a diverse clientele as it helps me to better myself by creating and adapting workouts to fit each individual. A lot of my clients work on the same goals but in different ways. As a trainer, I find it exciting to figure out what works best for each client.

15. What are the main benefits of working with a personal trainer?

For a lot of clients, it's the accountability that drives hiring a personal trainer. I would agree with that, but it also gives you someone to guide you towards your fitness goals. There is a lot of information on the internet and sifting through it can be quite burdensome. Having a good personal trainer will help you stay on track and should make workouts challenging and fun. Hiring a personal trainer is an investment in your overall health. Unlike a car or house, you only get one body.

Please tell us how readers can get in contact with you here:

Email: robertsb21@gmail.com

Website: musclebiology.wordpress.com

Twitter: @brob21

CHAPTER 7

HENRY HALSE

Please tell us about yourself and your company here:

Henry graduated from Ithaca College in 2014 with a degree in Clinical Exercise Science, which combines many different fields in exercise science and cardiac rehab training, using exercise to help someone recover from or prevent certain diseases. He is currently a certified personal trainer through the American College of Sports Medicine and a Certified Strength and Conditioning Specialist.

During his time at Ithaca, Henry completed three internships at different strength and conditioning facilities and worked as a personal trainer for staff and students for two years. While working as an intern at strength and conditioning gyms, Henry was able to train high school and college athletes, as well as assist in training MLB pitchers, NFL players, and MLS players.

Before coming to Philadelphia, Henry worked at Mike Boyle Strength and Conditioning in Boston, where he trained middle school, high school, college, and professional athletes. He also holds a volunteer position as a trainer at a rehabilitation program for men, where he uses exercise to teach self-discipline and helps others find strength to rebuild their lives.

Henry now owns Halse Strength and Fitness in Philadelphia and enjoys competing in powerlifting and learning as much as possible about the human body.

1. What is the best way to lose fat?

Fat is lost when that amount of calories consumed is less than the amount of calories used. This is called a negative energy balance. When your body stores fat, it is literally storing energy and each pound of fat contains about 3,000 calories. Therefore the only way to lose fat is to use more energy than you take in. This can be done by exercising, eating less, or a combination of the two. It's important to keep a steady rate of weight loss.

Do not try to lose more than 2 pounds per week. The goal is to lose fat but not muscle because muscle tissue is extremely active and will help you burn calories. Therefore, you should not be in a very high energy deficit. I suggest beginning an exercise program and sticking to it for a while (at least a year) before you really start to cut back on your food intake. This is because you will not want to start exercising while you are reducing your food intake because you will have less energy. Start with exercise and focus on eating habits later. When you finally feel you are ready to work on nutrition, make sure that you track the calorie and macronutrient content of the food you eat. It will be difficult to change your eating habits if you don't even know what they are! What are the chances that you can remember what you had for dinner last Tuesday? Start to write it down and you will begin to notice patterns in your diet that you might want to change. Another thing to consider with rapid weight loss is that your metabolism will slow down if you drop the amount of calories you eat too quickly. When your metabolism drops you are no longer expending energy quickly and it will be much tougher to lose fat. That is why exercise is more effective than diet for fat loss. You can simply add more exercise or make it more intense in order to burn more calories. Do not make rapid changes to your diet or it will come back to bite you.

2. I have an event coming up in 2 months. What's my best strategy for getting in better shape by then?

In order to get in shape quickly, you will need to jump into an exercise program. Focus on exercises that are simple and have a low risk of injury. If you need to be in shape in two months the best option would be to combine weight training and interval training into a circuit. For example: squat for 10 reps, jump rope for 30 seconds, as many push-ups as you can, then 10 burpees. This way you are getting the benefits of weight training and cardio in the same workout. If you really need help with your eating habits, it would be wise to contact a registered dietician who can give you expert advice that will bypass all of the trial and error of dieting.

Make sure that you don't pursue your goal too aggressively-avoid sickness and injury at all costs! Both of them are symptoms of too much stress so make sure that you don't push too hard. If you get sick or injured, then you can't train and that is the worst setback of all.

3. Is walking or running better for fat loss?

According to an energy expenditure calculator, a 200lb person would burn 726 calories running at 5mph for an hour but only burn 270 calories from walking at 2mph for an hour. That's a difference of almost 500 calories!

And 5mph is a slow run! Walking is one of the most biomechanically efficient activities that humans do. In fact, one could argue that we were built to walk long distances without consuming much energy. When humans walk, we basically fall onto the leg in front of us and then are carried by that leg until the other leg reaches the ground in front. Instead of propelling ourselves forward we are essentially constantly falling forward, which is incredibly efficient. Therefore, running is absolutely better for fat loss because it burns more calories!

4. Should I do cardio or weight training?

Weight training can raise your resting metabolic rate (the amount of energy you use while not exercising) for up to 48 hours while running will only increase it for about 3 hours. That is a massive difference! Especially considering that you will probably burn more calories from your metabolism doing its job than from exercise in a given day. Weight training also encourages muscle growth, which is extremely active metabolic tissue. More muscle mass requires more energy, therefore increasing your metabolic rate. One of the easiest ways to lose fat is to build up your resting metabolic rate because you will be able to lose more fat without doing anything!

Just keep in mind that weight training is more difficult than cardio as far as technique goes, so make sure you have someone show you how to properly use the weights.

5. What are your recommended workouts for fast results?

For someone looking to get generally fit a mix of weights and cardio in a circuit, format is the best. Alternate a strength exercise with a cardiovascular exercise. The same example I used in a previous question still applies: squat, jump rope, push-up, and burpee. When you combine strength and cardio in a circuit you can get the benefit of both types of exercises and you can get your workout done in a reasonable amount of time as opposed to breaking strength and cardio into two different workouts. It is important to note that there is a law of diminishing returns with exercise. Doing one set of an exercise will be good, two might be better, three might be optimal. Beyond that, your returns start to diminish. Four sets may be a little better than three but not by much. Five sets may be almost the same as four. Therefore you should workout as much as you have to in order to get results, but not more. Your body can only adapt at a certain speed and it will take time.

6. How can I speed up my recovery period?

Sleep, calories, carbohydrates, and stress management are the big four. If you lack, any of these your ability to recover will be compromised. Massage, ice baths, and supplements may all play a role in recovery, but they are not nearly as important as the big four. Sleep is first and foremost because reductions in performance have been seen after only a few days of reduced sleep.

7. How often should I workout?

The amount of high-intensity workouts in a week should restricted because those are the workouts that will really take a toll on your body. I recommend starting with two really high-intensity workouts per week and then after a month add another high-intensity workout. You should be active every single day. This means going on walks as often as possible, doing light exercises or less intense exercise classes such as yoga. Human beings were made to be active all day so make sure that you are moving around as much as possible. You want to have the mentality of a hyperactive child, always moving and energetic. This keeps your energy expenditure higher throughout the day. Start slow with the very intense workouts but be active as much as possible.

8. How do I get a flat stomach?

The short answer is simply to lose fat in the ways that we have discussed. Make sure that you lose the fat in a slow and sustainable way if you would like to keep it off. Something else that people don't discuss is bloating. If you eat something that you don't digest well, your stomach will bloat and stick out more than you would like. Be conscious of the way that different meals make you feel and if your stomach sticks out more after eating certain foods. Then you will know what to avoid in the future if you have an event coming up. You can do ab workouts but they won't really mean much until you lose the fat that lies on top of the abs.

9. How do I get rid of flabby arms?

This simply comes down to losing fat. Spot reduction is not possible and honestly doing arm exercises is a waste of time if you are trying to lose fat. You should spend time doing lower body exercises and some high-intensity circuits. You can do some arms to build up muscle, but you won't be able to see that muscle until you lose fat.

10. What short workouts can I do between work?

It's important to get moving during your lunch break to keep your energy levels up. At the very least get out and walk somewhere to get your blood flowing. You can also throw in some bodyweight squats, push-ups, lunges, and planks for a little more difficulty. Another option is to find some stairs to walk up and down for about 20 minutes. You will find that the more you exercise during the day, the more energy you have!

11. What is the best diet to follow?

The best diet to follow is the one that allows you to eat foods that you enjoy and makes you feel the best. If the diet that you are on tells you to eat certain types of foods, then it will not work! The most important thing is consistency. It is by far more important than the type of food that you eat. Some people try very restrictive diets such as a low carb diet. If you think that you can live the rest of your life on a low carbohydrate diet then go for it, but I don't believe that anyone would willingly do that to themselves. There is no additional benefit to restricting one macronutrient either. The only thing that matters is calories in vs. calories out. 100 calories from a cookie is the same as 100 calories from broccoli. Calories are simply a unit of energy. Therefore, the best diet to follow is a diet that you enjoy but a diet that you track on a calorie counter and monitor. That way you can set a calorie limit and then decide how you reach that limit. This is the easiest way to be consistent and therefore the best way to diet.

12. Do I need to take dietary supplements?

If there is a deficiency in your diet that you can't fix with food then take supplements. Sometimes it is cheaper to take a supplement than to buy the food that contains equal amounts of the substance. A good example is fish oil, since fish can be very expensive to buy in large quantities. Other than that supplements are a gigantic waste of money. That is why the supplement industry is worth billions of dollars! They are just trying to make money off of you.

13. What tips do you have for healthy food on the go?

The easiest way to eat healthy on the go is to make food at home and bring it in Tupperware. You can also buy granola or protein bars that you like and bring them with you. This gives you the most control over the food that you are eating. If you need to go to a restaurant you can plan it out in advance and find something that looks agreeable, but there is much less control. You don't know how they are cooking your food, if it is cooked in fat or butter, how much salt is in it, etc.

14. Who is your ideal client to work with?

Someone who wants to be a part of the process. This means that they ask questions about what we are doing and why and they are willing to work hard. When someone starts to become more involved in their training it is a sign that they will be successful. Those are the people that ask what they can be doing outside of the gym to improve even more. This is the ultimate form of motivation, where I don't even have to push them because they are motivated by themselves. I can only control what someone does for two or three hours per week in the gym, but your fitness goals need to be pursued 24/7. I really enjoy watching these people progress and I know that even if they leave my gym that they will keep improving.

15. What are the main benefits of working with a personal trainer?

It's the same as with any other profession. I don't do my own taxes because I want to know that they are being done correctly and I don't know enough to do them perfectly. If you are looking to get into working out, you should contact a professional so that you can do it safely and effectively. I never had a personal trainer as a kid and I made a lot of mistakes while I tried to figure out what worked. I could have saved years of toiling in the gym with little to no success by hiring a trainer. It is worth the money because you don't have to work with a trainer for the rest of your life, only long enough to learn how to properly exercise. Personal trainers are just exercise professionals, so if you need exercise advice that is who you should go to.

Please tell us how readers can get in contact with you here:

Email: robertsb21@gmail.com

Website: www.halsesf.com

Facebook: Halse Strength and Fitness

Instagram: halsesf

CHAPTER 8

ERIK CLINE

Please tell us about yourself here:

I am a Certified Life Coach. I help eager individuals navigate the complicated jungles of life both personally and professionally. I work both one on one and in groups in a very empowering process, to raise client awareness, move past barriers, expedite change, and achieve goals. My goal for each client is their optimal success and fulfillment, or their maximum potential.

My mission is to provide a high level of positive, inspiring Coaching to improve people's personal and professional lives. I apply my vast experience, education and training - along with my unique coaching style- to move people seeking change and fulfillment. I help people advance in their lives by successfully achieving their goals. My aim with each client is their maximum potential or happiness, no matter what their intention may be. My style is a blend of empathy, and fun yet always being firm in pushing my clients.

1. What is the best way to lose fat?

Simply by burning more energy than consumed over a given period of time. This is much easier said than done. For most people, it will involve a mixture of diet, exercise, and adequate rest.

2. I have an event coming up in 2 months. What's my best strategy for getting in better shape by then?

Take some time to analyze your normal diet and daily habits to figure out what needs to be changed. Define your goal and begin to develop a plan. A great idea is to implement a document of sorts. A journal, calendar, spreadsheet, or post it note, whatever will work for you to make your plan tangible. Also sharing your plan with others (friends, family, social media, etc.) to help keep you accountable for the defined goal. Then begin working towards the goal. Make diet changes if needed, and increase, or change up the exercise routine. Track your progress, and utilize any help or opportunity along the way.

Keep up with the journal or accountability partners. Also take some time to plan for obstacles, or complications along the way, to better combat them when they arise.

3. Is walking or running better for fat loss?

Running is better for fat loss as it usually gets the heart rate higher, resulting in more energy being burnt. But if one cannot run for any reason, walking is still a good way to get moving. As long as it is briskly and with an increased heart rate, one could see results. Walking steep hills or hiking is good for fat loss when running is not an option.

4. Should I do cardio or weight training?

Both. Complete fitness comes from a mixture of both. But the two can be done simultaneously, assuming the choice of workout. And weight training can be done with just body weight. One can achieve very solid workout routines with minimal or no equipment at home. Cardio or weight training, no gym required.

5. What are your recommended workouts for fast results?

High-intensity interval training. Pushing one's limits for a short time followed by even shorter periods of rest and repeating. Like the famed Tabata workout, where one works as fast as possible for 20 seconds followed by 10 seconds rest. This is repeated 8 times for a total of 4 minutes. When done with say 4 different movements the result is a very effective 16-minute workout. There are many different apps and lots of internet content to assist in getting started with these types of workouts.

Movements can include: pushups, squats, pullups, planks, situps and crunches. Or light weight lifting or jumping rope. The fun comes in changing up the movements or adding more sets, also in tracking results and working to improve times and reps.

Calisthenics like pushups or pull ups and static holds like planks that focus on heavy core utilization are great to boost the metabolism, promoting weight loss.

Also workouts that involve a lot of different body parts, such as swimming, pilates, and certain types of yoga can get fast results when done with the right level of strenuousness.

For fast results, workouts must feel uncomfortable. If it's too easy then it's time to change it up. Faster speeds, longer distances, heavier weight, or more reps. Exercise that is too easy will not likely get fast results. Results come from getting uncomfortable, and that "uncomfort" can be in the way you exercise, the things you eat, and getting a good nights sleep. Big leaps in progress occur when we find ease in the things that were once uncomfortable.

6. How can I speed up my recovery period?

Immediately after workout- focus on breath recovery. Breathing is a very overlooked part of fitness and is crucial. Deep breathing exercises can help this. Shortly after workout- hydration, healthy food/energy replacement. Also stretching and massage, and rest or good sleep.

7. How often should I workout?

Almost daily. Whether its for a few minutes or few hours. Even if it's just some light stretching for a bit, or a short walk. Few of our days should be spent being stationary.

8. How do I get a flat stomach?

By burning fat calories, and increasing muscle. Fat is not burnt in one area of the body, it is lost throughout the entire body at once. A common myth is that fat can be lost in one area of focus, but this is not so. Building the muscles of the upper body can help create a slimmer look, and the muscle mass also helps in boosting metabolism, which in turn can lead to that coveted flat stomach.The only way that I know of to remove fat in one area of the body is through invasive medical procedures.

9. How do I get rid of flabby arms?

Same as the flabby stomach. Burning fat calories all over the body and increasing muscle mass, especially in the upper arm area in this case.

10. What short workouts can I do between work?

High-intensity interval or Tabata style workouts, where maximum effort is given for short times(usually 30 seconds or less) followed by short rest periods(20 seconds or less) from a few minutes to a half hour at most. These bodyweight workout circuits (push ups, pull ups, squats, planks, etc.) are great as they can be done almost anywhere, with little or no equipment.

If you're looking to breakup they workday with small bits of exercise, the high-intensity workouts can be a bit much. It's never fun to sweat profusely and go back to working. But short sets of things like squats or pushups or pullups can be done without too much sweat breaking. A good way to stay strong and build muscle throughout the work day, without needing to shower. Maybe a set of 20 pushups once or twice and hour through the day. These add up, and make the harder workouts easier over time. I recommend keeping some deodorant in the car or desk, though.

11. What is the best diet to follow?

As close to natural and as far from processed as possible. No particular diet is best, but with the proper knowledge of what we are putting into our bodies we can better control how we will look, feel, and perform. You are what you eat. Whatever the diet is, it should be rich in lean protein, and vitamins from edible plants. Low in bleached or processed carbs, little or no sugar added, and void of preservatives, artificial color, and chemicals.

12. Do I need to take dietary supplements?

Not if your diet is ideal. But an ideal diet is tough to achieve, so supplements can provide what is lacking. Proper evaluation of diet and understanding of what is lacking, is necessary to choosing the right supplements.

13. What tips do you have for healthy food on the go?

Fruit, vegetables, nuts, granola. Juices and smoothies can be a great way to pack in nutrients quickly and on the go. Portability is key for many who stay on a solid diet. Packing food to bring is a huge plus. Plastic containers and bags, with healthy foods, is great for on the go people. It is good practice to cook and prepare food to bring ahead of time, making for easy grab and go in our ever busy world.

14. Who is your ideal client to work with?

Someone who knows what they want for themselves, and is ready to work past the excuses and push for results. Future focused individuals who are ready and willing to make changes, and embrace uncomfort.

15. What are the main benefits of working with a personal trainer?

Learning the correct exercise techniques, from someone with experience who knows how to minimize injury. Having someone to push you and celebrate exercise milestones with. Also having a partner for accountability.

Please tell us how readers can get in contact with you here:

Email: coach@erikcline.com

Phone: 631-637-1272

Facebook, Twitter, Linkedin, Instagram: @coacherikcline

CHAPTER 9

TREVA BRANDON SCHARF

Please tell us about yourself here:

I am a Los Angeles based personal fitness trainer and group fitness instructor with over 30 years of experience working with classes and private clients. My unique system of cross training includes core conditioning, traditional resistance training, coaching, and functional fitness. It burns fat, builds muscle, and gets results.

1. What is the best way to lose fat?

The best way to lose fat is to cut down on calorie intake and increase cardiovascular exercise. There is no magic bullet, powder, supplement, or miracle juice cleanse, I'm sorry to say. It's being smart with your diet, disciplined in your exercise, committed to your goals, and reasonable in your expectations. The bottom line? Do the work and you'll get results.

2. I have an event coming up in 2 months. What's my best strategy for getting in better shape by then?

For fast results, I'd recommend drastically reducing carbs, not eating after 6 pm, eliminating alcohol temporarily, and upping your workouts to 3x a week.

3. Is walking or running better for fat loss?

Not everyone is cut out for running, but everyone, for the most part, can walk. If you can run, run. But if you're walking, make sure it's at a brisk pace for at least 30 minutes. And make it challenging - include hills, trails, speed work, etc. Mix it up and make it interesting. Scenery, music, audiobook, whatever it takes to keep you engaged and moving.

4. Should I do cardio or weight training?

By all means do both! Cardio combined with traditional resistance training leads to excellent conditioning, increased muscle mass, and improved stamina and endurance. Especially if you're over 50, I'd suggest a program of weights and cardio for heart disease prevention and bone density.

5. What are your recommended workouts for fast results?

I love any kind of hybrid exercise that combines agility, coordination, and dynamic balance. Bootcamp, TRX, CrossFit, sculpt classes, stair running, anything that will amp up your metabolism.

6. How can I speed up my recovery period?

The most overlooked part of any smart exercise program is REST. It's as important as the workout itself. Don't be afraid to take a day or two off. Make sure you stay hydrated, include massage therapy and stretching into your recovery, and practice meditation. Your mind and body will thank you.

7. How often should I workout?

Work out as much as you like, or as much as your body can handle. Mixing up your workouts with different equipment and routines not only helps spare your body excessive wear and tear, but it also prevents boredom from setting in. For this reason, I like cross training - it allows you to work many different muscle groups without burning you out.

8. How do I get a flat stomach?

Unless you're in your 20s, or are a body builder, or are genetically lean, or love starvation diets, it's very difficult to get a flat stomach. Add in age and hormones, and it gets even more impossible. I've never seen anyone over 30-years-old with a six-pack unless they're getting paid to look that way. Keeping your body fat low will accentuate all your muscles, including your abs. Increasing core work will help build ab definition, but you can't "sit-up" your way to a flat stomach.

9. How do I get rid of flabby arms?

As I mentioned, keeping your body fat low by eating a lean diet helps define all your muscles, including arms. Upper body weight training and swimming are two of the most effective forms of arm work you can do to build strength and tighten things up. However, with age and other factors (sun damage, smoking, etc.), skin just naturally loses it elasticity over time. Yes, it sucks, but what can I say? Mother Nature is a bitch sometimes.

10. What short workouts can I do between work?

Bring your sneakers to work and take a brisk walk at lunch time. Or, if you have more time and belong to a gym, a 45-minute indoor cycling class would do the trick.

11. What is the best diet to follow?

There is no "best diet" to follow. It's called using your head and eating smart. Fill your diet with as much fresh produce as possible, meat and carbs are ok in small amounts. Stay away from fried and processed foods, or products that have too many ingredients on the label. As for alcohol, desserts, and the occasional pizza? Moderation all the way.

12. Do I need to take dietary supplements?

Not unless it's for medical reasons and your doctor prescribes them, I say no to supplements. It's a waste of time, money, and a total scam perpetrated on the American public.

13. What tips do you have for healthy food on the go?

Keep pre-filled baggies of trail mix, nuts, or fresh fruit in your car, in your desk, or in your purse. It will stave off hunger until you're able to sit down and have a proper meal.

14. Who is your ideal client to work with?

My ideal client is serious. They're not there to fuck around. Whether they're young, old, a former athlete, or sedentary for years, a good client is someone who is disciplined, committed, and goal oriented. They show up, they do the work, and they don't complain.

15. What are the main benefits of working with a personal trainer?

You can be an elite athlete or overweight blob, it doesn't matter. A trainer is great for everyone, of any level. A good trainer will push you beyond your limits; inspire you to achieve more; help work through your fears, and love and support you when no one else will.

Please tell us how readers can get in contact with you here:

treva@trevabrandonscharf.com

CHAPTER 10

MARIE DELCIOPPO & LAUREN MANISCALCO

Please tell us about your company here:

Marie is a New York Times featured Raw Foods Chef, Health Coach, Pilates Instructor, Personal Trainer, Strategic Marketing Consultant for Lifestyle Brands and Health + Wellness Entrepreneurs.

Lauren Maniscalco, the owner and founder of Coastal Body Studio. She opened Coastal Body Studio in Charleston, SC, originally just offering Pilates and nutritional counseling. But staying on the cutting edge of fitness and wellness and challenging her clients to the next level, she has since introduced Barre, Yoga, Physical Therapy, Massage, Nutrition, and doTerra Essential Oils.

1. What is the best way to lose fat?

FOR EXERCISE:

High-intensity Interval Training (HIIT) will give you some serious bang for your fitness buck.

What Is HIIT?

HIIT is any workout that alternates between intense bursts

of activity and recovery (either a fixed period of less-intense activity or even complete rest).

Ideally done two to three times a week, HIIT workouts last a MAX of thirty minutes so they are an excellent choice when you're crunched for time. A measly fifteen minutes of HIIT (done three times a week) is more effective than jogging for sixty minutes.

There are many benefits to HIIT, aside from the time saving.

First, many HIIT workouts combine strength (predominantly movements working multiple muscle groups at the same time to spike your heart rate) and cardio moves, meaning you sculpt muscle tone while you blast fat.

And anyone who's tried to lose weight knows how hard it is to lose fat without also losing muscle. Studies show that HIIT allow dieters to lose the fat and keep their hard earned muscle tone.

In addition to increased fat burning and more muscle development and preservation, HIIT stimulates the production of human growth hormone (HGH) by up to 450% in the twenty-four hours post workout. HGH is responsible for increased calorie burn and slowing the aging process, keeping you looking young inside and out.

As a bonus, not only do you burn more calories during a HIIT workout than during an endurance workout, but you also continue to burn more calories and fat for twenty-four hours post-workout.

Finally, you can do a HIIT workout anywhere, anytime because there's no special equipment required. Run, high knees, jumping jacks, mountain climbers, jumping lunges, burpees...

These all make for a great HIIT session. In fact, dumbbells can make a HIIT workout less effective because your goal in HIIT is to focus on pushing your heart rate — not your biceps — to the max.

FOR FOOD:

Personally I like to see people eliminate sugar (and all of the secret names it goes by like those listed here http://lushvitality. com/death-by-sugar/), gluten, alcohol, caffeine, dairy, and many soy products for 30 days. As I had mentioned in another response, these are the most common food intolerances and metabolize as acidic, which means they lead to inflammation and can pack on the pounds and make it difficult to lose weight. I actually lead a 30 day cleanse and restore program where we eliminate these foods and also provide not only gut and liver cleansing but also restoration and proper supplementation (http://lushvitality.com/30-day-cleanse-restore-program/).

However, all of that being said, many times people find it more practical to have a basic guideline to follow. When I talk about eliminating anything that's white, I'm referring to refined sugar and flour (even those labeled "whole wheat" and "sugar in the raw" are nothing more than highly processed flour and sugar with food coloring added to appear more "natural") and table salt. Salts like Himalayan (pink) and Celtic Sea Salt (gray) are loaded with trace minerals and actually beneficial to you and don't send your sodium soaring. What I want people to focus on is trashing the processed foods that are loaded with the "white" foods - refined sugar, flour, and salt - and even those highly pasteurized and processed cheeses and dairy products.

You often hear that it's a good idea to shop the perimeter of the grocery, and this is true! You want to load your cart with produce (organic whenever possible) and, if you do choose to eat animal products, wild game, free range, organic foul and eggs, and wild caught, low mercury fishes. And you can still do sweets! Dates, molasses, and using stevia (but not white!) moderately are all excellent low-glycemic options. Obviously we don't want these making up the majority of our calories, but for a treat, these are wonderful because they also have fiber and molasses is an excellent source of potassium and iron. I also recommend 100% pure Grade B maple syrup and raw agave to use on occasion because they are not as highly processed and, like the others, do not spike our blood sugar.

I want people to load up on good white food like coconut and cauliflower!

Also, when we think about exercising, if you do an endurance workout — a 45-minute run, for example — you blow out your glycogen stores. This means you're more likely to get extremely hungry and crave sugar and carbs. Plus, with a workout like HIIT, you're increasing your muscle mass, which, in turn, revs your metabolism.

2. I have an event coming up in 2 months. What's my best strategy for getting in better shape by then?

Plan on working out five to six times a week. Three of those workouts will be HIIT workouts and the other two to three should be something no nonsense, like a 60-minute advanced Pilates, Barre, or other high-intensity class that focuses on proper body mechanics and sculpting while still elevating your heart rate.

Look into doing a 30-day detox program where you are cleansing and then restoring your liver and gut. This is not a starvation program! You will eat. You will focus on eliminating gluten, dairy, alcohol, caffeine, sugar, and many soy products, as these are the most common food intolerances and highly inflammatory, acid forming foods. The program should be led by a qualified nutritionist or health coach and include proper supplements as well as strict guidance. You and your coach should work one-on-one to make sure you are eating properly and not going into starvation mode.

The second month you can then begin to reintroduce foods so when you show up to your event, you don't binge on the cheese platter and unravel it all.

3. Is walking or running better for fat loss?

Whichever one you'll actually get up off the couch and do is the one that's better.

Keep in mind: If you are walking or running at a less intense pace, you will want to go for a longer duration.

4. Should I do cardio or weight training?

Ideally you're integrating both like you do with HIIT.

When we see people with a lot of weight to loose, we often start them with just cardio to get the weight off and to get them used to moving. And often they are not agile enough to do an effective strength training routine. But they can definitely go for a walk! If you're within 20 pounds of your ideal weight, you need to add in strength training in order to help with proper body alignment (which in and of itself can burn hundreds more calories per day) and increased muscle mass, both of which fuel your metabolism.

5. What are your recommended workouts for fast results?

HIIT and Barre.

Barre is an excellent overall sculpting and toning workout. It combines elements of resistance training (using light weights, bands, and balls), Pilates, Ballet, and calisthenics. It is high-intensity without being high impact, so it's excellent on your joints and for those recovering from injury or who may be working through one. Like Pilates, your instructor can offer you a variety of modifications, so no matter what your level, you can get a killer workout.

You will do movements like push-ups, planks, and dips. And your heart rate will elevate because of the large muscle compound movements — there is a long leg section in Barre class so you get serious lower body sculpting. In fact, most class patrons say their lower body has never looked better than when they do barre on a regular basis.

There is a strong emphasis on alignment, so you train your body to be in excellent posture while chiseling long, lean muscle tone.

I often say it resembles Pilates but standing. Many of the same elements and principles but standing to really get that effect of gravity to challenge you further.

What's unique about Barre is the use of the ballet barre for many of the movements. However, if you were to do at home workouts, you can use the back of a chair or a countertop.

6. How can I speed up my recovery period?

Log 7-8 hours of deep restorative sleep per night.

Properly hydrate by drinking a minimum of half your body weight in ounces of water per day.

Stretch.

Eat high-quality complete proteins, meaning they have all nine essential amino acids. Don't be as concerned about the grams of protein a food contains as you are about it being a complete protein from a clean (organic) source.

7. How often should I workout?

Five to six days a week for thirty to sixty minutes per workout session.

8. How do I get a flat stomach?

You have to loose weight. There's no getting around it. You can have strong core muscles, but they can be hidden under a layer of fat.

Also focus on core strengthening — not just crunches but all over core training with something like Pilates. What's going to pull your stomach in is a proper balance of strength and flexibility between your abdominals, back, inner thighs, and shoulders. Just getting people to stand in proper alignment can make it look like they instantly lost ten pounds.

9. How do I get rid of flabby arms?

Just as with the stomach, you have to lose the fat. No amount of toning exercises will help when there's a lot of fat. That being said, if you are within your target weight range or just slightly above, you can improve the tone of your upper body with exercises like push-ups and tricep dips.

10. What short workouts can I do between work?

Take the stairs, park further away from the front door, do squats and lunges holding onto your desk or back of your chair, do tricep dips on your office chair and incline push-ups with your hands on the desk. Do one minute of jump rope or jumping jacks so you don't get super sweaty and do that several times throughout the day. When you are sitting and even standing, reinforce good posture — feel as though you are zipping up your tightest pair of pants, buttoning a tight shirt, and let your shoulders fall, feeling all that tension melt down your back.

11. What is the best diet to follow?

No processed foods, lots of dark, leafy greens, alkaline, predominantly plant-based, and organic. If you are going to eat animal products, steer clear of dairy, but you can do organic and free-range foul, wild game, and wild caught, low mercury fish like salmon, mackerel, halibut, and sardines in moderation (two to three times per week.

12. Do I need to take dietary supplements?

Yes. First, you want a whole food, bioavailable vitamin and mineral supplement that has a balanced profile of vitamins and minerals (no mega doses) and trace minerals. Then you want an essential fatty acid formula with either clean fish sources like sardines or plant sources like flax and hemp. In addition, you want to take a probiotic in a double layer capsule so it is not released until it hits your intestines as well as a digestive enzyme complex.

13. What tips do you have for healthy food on the go?

Apples, pears, berries, goji berries, raisins, raw (unroasted and unsalted) nuts and seeds, hummus, avocado, sliced veggies. Always have snacks and your water bottle on hand so you don't find yourself ravenous at pulling into the nearest drive through. Also, many times we confuse thirst for hunger, so make sure you have water with you at all times and that you're actually drinking it.

14. Who is your ideal client to work with?

The one who is open to learning and receptive to feedback. Who is honest with themselves about where they are versus where they want to be and is willing to do the work to get there. Who has a good attitude and doesn't whine and complain. Who realizes being in prime health is what will give them quality of life and success in all areas.

15. What are the main benefits of working with a personal trainer?

You will see results faster with a trainer because she is watching your form and will not leave any room for you to slack off. The difference between doing an exercise to its maximum potential and with even the slightest improper form can be the difference between injury and not and even make the difference in the number of calories you burn, so a trained professional eye is critical.

Then there's also the fact that you're paying someone. You're accountable. If you don't show up, you still have to pay for the session.

Please tell us how readers can get in contact with you here:

Marie Delcioppo, Owner, Lush Vitality

(786) 359-3070

marie@lushvitality.com

www.lushvitality.com

Lauren Maniscalco, Owner, Coastal Body Studio

(843) 801-3939

Lauren@CoastalBody.com

www.CoastalBody.com

CHAPTER 11

MARISA SILVER

Please tell us about your company here:

In The Zone Personal Fitness is a private training facility on Long Island, NY. We pride ourselves on providing our clients with the productive fitness training one can have in 30 minutes. Our clients range from the professional athletes to the 65-year-old that wants to lose 25 lbs. Our trainers are certified, experienced and have a passion to help others achieve their goals.

1. What is the best way to lose fat?

If I had to ask myself what is the number one question I get asked every day, it would be "how do I lose fat"...

I tell my clients that losing weight/fat is a simple math equation. We have all taken math but for some reason, when it comes to understanding calories, people are confused and dumbfounded on how to begin. What most people don't understand, is that to maintain a certain weight you have to be consuming enough calories to maintain what it reads on the scale. People have said to me, that no matter what they do or how they eat, they are unable to lose weight.

In order to lose weight, one has to burn more Calories than consumed. 3500 Calories equals one pound.

In order to lose one pound per week, one would have to eliminate 500 Calories a day. The best way to accomplish this is to consume lower Calorie food choices or smaller servings in combination with exercise.

For example: Decrease your intake by 250 Calories and burn 250 Calories per day. This is an easier method than just reducing 500 Calories a day by dietary restrictions or trying to burn off 500 Calories per day.

2. I have an event coming up in 2 months. What's my best strategy for getting in better shape by then?

When someone has an event coming up it always makes it easier as a trainer to put a regimen together. People are more inclined to follow a plan if they know that there is an end date. To begin with, I always suggest with a simple walk around the block. From there you can start to walk half the block and alternate between running and walking. If this is done every other day you will not only see a decrease in weight loss but in an increase in tone and stamina. Next, of course, is food. It's a question of eating healthy and portion control. If you have an event and it means "discipline" watch those calories and fat grams. Eat 5-6 managed portions and cut out the empty calorie snacking. I always saw when it comes to snacking do not eat anything that comes in a bag!! Have fruits or yogurt to snack on. Keep a journal so you can see how the food you eat affects your mood and please buy a scale and weight in once a week in the morning. I suggest hiring a personal trainer and set aside two-three times a week in which you would dedicate your time to fitness training. Have your trainer show you exercises that you can do on your off days at home to help facilitate your weight loss and getting in shape.

3. Is walking or running better for fat loss?

Walking and running are very popular among people that are trying to lose weight or stay in shape. Running is obviously more strenuous then walking and, therefore, would burn more calories. People that walk tend to exercise longer than people that run. On the other hand, people who begin to walk rather than run when they are starting a weight loss regimen are probably older and more unhealthy than those who just started running. Either way, you can't go wrong when you start to exercise. But if you have no previous joint injuries and you are in fairly decent shape, I would start to jog as a happy medium to lose fat, tone muscles and increase your cardiovascular health.

4. Should I do cardio or weight training?

I believe that both cardio and weight training have to be done in order to achieve maximum results. The essential goals are core strengthening, stamina, and weight loss. Weight training alone will increase your muscularity. It will increase the strength of tendons, build strength and help with osteoporosis. The benefits of cardiovascular fitness training are weight loss, enhancing heart muscle fitness and lung capacity. The benefits of doing both together outweigh doing one without the other.

5. What are your recommended workouts for fast results?

. To get quick results, you should train an hour every day. These workouts should be cardio based. That means in addition to weight training you are also adding an element of cardio at the same time. For example, instead of doing a deep squats you are doing a higher jump squat. Instead of doing a bicep curl, you are performing your curls with an added lunge. Always trying to incorporate two moves at the same time to get the maximum benefit of each movement. If you have an event coming up and you want to look your best, I recommend doing cardio alone such as jogging for 30 min a day in addition to your cardio based workout. Let's not forget and the abdominal musculature. Adding crunches to your regimen will flatten your stomach and increase your core strength allowing you to run further and exercise longer.

6. How can I speed up my recovery period?

A light cardio workout can decrease your recovery time and help to remove some of the by-products that were created during the weight training session. This will help reduce the delayed onset of muscle soreness. Another added benefit is bringing oxygenated blood to the muscle to improve in building and repair. Your body is built to heal from the inside out so nutrition can play an important role in the recovery period. Foods to include are ones rich in Vitamin C: citrus, berries, peppers, and broccoli. Vitamin A: Carrots, sweet potatoes, and spinach. Omega 3: salmon, flax seeds, and walnuts. Zinc: oysters, nuts, seeds and chicken.

7. How often should I workout?

A person should consider fitness and health as a lifestyle, not a temporary chore. A consistent fitness regimen can vary from a light walk around the block to a more intense training session. One can do a moderate cardiovascular workout every day. You can also do light strength training every day. On the other hand, if the workout is strenuous on your individual muscles and joints then I suggest alternating body parts and giving your body one day a week to rest and heal.

8. How do I get a flat stomach?

In order to attain a flat stomach two things must be incorporated, a cardiovascular exercise routine to burn calories and an abdominal workout. People forget that the abdominal musculature are like any other muscles in the body. In order to develop the muscles, they must be used. This can be accomplished by doing crunches and sit-ups. I only recommend sit-ups to clients that have had no previous back injuries or trauma. For the beginner I recommend crunches. This is an exercise that can be done every day. I recommend 25 per day and then gradually build up from there.

9. How do I get rid of flabby arms?

My preference is to exercise with 3-5 lb. weights to develop definition. Anything more than that will cause your muscles to appear more bulky with less muscle definition. I recommend 2 sets of 12 repetitions of bicep curls and 2 sets of 12 repetitions of tricep push backs. I think the deltoid muscle is just as important as it is the muscle that encompasses the shoulder and can be seen in every direction. I also recommend deltoid raises in anterior, medial and posterior directions for development. Of course, it is equally important to have a low caloric diet so that the muscles striations show rather than a puffy look of extra adipose tissue.

10. What short workouts can I do between work?

Work days can be long, I recommend that my clients walk during their lunch break. It's a great way to de- stress and burn some added calories. If you are fortunate enough to have a private office you can always bring in a yoga matt and perform pushups during a break. Even tricep lifts can be done on a desk. Lunges can also be done while waiting for the phone to ring or sending a fax.

11. What is the best diet to follow?

I don't like the word diet. I feel that word comes with a beginning and an ending. When someone wants to start a journey for health it should never have an ending. A lifestyle of low carbohydrates and fats is essential for healthy living. It is important incorporate lots of fruits and vegetables and suggest eating 5-6 small meals a day. This is not only a good way to remain satisfied, but you would be less likely to binge. It will help keep your sugar and energy levels even throughout the day and prevent the highs and lows that most people suffer when they eat less often during the day.

12. Do I need to take dietary supplements?

I do believe in dietary supplements such as vitamins and minerals. Unfortunately due to our busy lifestyles, the majority of people are not getting the proper amount of fruits and vegetables in their diet. We are also very aware of the sun and the damage that it can do to our skin. It is very common to have a vitamin D deficiency. I don't believe in supplements for weight loss, I think they are dangerous and many of the dangers are unfortunately not known yet.

13. What tips do you have for healthy food on the go?

We are very fortunate that it is easier to eat healthy snacks now than ever before. There are many prepacked snakes at our disposal. You can get raisins, almonds, nuts, carrots, apple slices, granola bars, plus many other healthy snacks that come prepackaged for our convenience. I like making my own with raisins, yogurt raisins, almonds, and cranberries. I suggest making these low calorie "to go" packs the night before. Apples, bananas, pears are also a great source for food on the go. Always remember to plan ahead so you don't feel the urge to stop off at a convenient drive through to satisfy your need for lack of planning.

14. Who is your ideal client to work with?

My ideal client is someone that is honest about their goals.

It's discouraging when you meet a client and they give you a deadline for weight loss, especially with unrealistic expectations. It's important to understand that it has taken some time to put on extra weight or become unhealthy. A few training sessions are not going to reverse the process. It takes hard work and dedication. If a client walks in my door understanding these concepts, then I know we will succeed together in achieving their goals.

15. What are the main benefits of working with a personal trainer?

There are many benefits of hiring a personal trainer. One of best benefits, you get a built in cheering section. You have someone watching and coaching you throughout your workout. Not only will a trainer change the workout and advance you when needed, your trainer will spot the client and prevent injury. I have many clients train on their own on equipment that either they did not know how to use or they used improper weight that caused them injury. If someone is serious about fitness and taking it to the next level, a personal trainer is essential.

Please tell us how readers can get in contact with you here:

Readers can find us at our website: www.bodybysilver.com

In the Zone Personal Fitness

62 Bethpage Road

Hicksville, NY 11801

516-216-4279

CHAPTER 12

ILARIA CAVAGNA

Please tell us about your company here:

Vogue hi-lighted instructor Ilaria Cavagna combines her knowledge of Pilates, Soma Training, Myofascial stretching and Eldoa to better the lives of her clients. Her philosophy is to partner with each client to find an enjoyable, sustainable and hard working path to their goals.

In addition to her "one on one" training, Ilaria is an international presenter of health and wellness workshops in Chile, Italy, Spain and here in the United States. She works by Skype as well to help trainers break through the plateaus all clients eventually encounter.

Ilaria is developing a revolutionary approach to women's wellness for release along with her book in 2016.

1. What is the best way to lose fat?

What is the best way to lose fat? We all know that losing fat is not a matter of doing one thing only, but rather it's a process. On top of that, while the energy we introduce and the activity we execute may be the same, the results will vary based on factors such as activity background, health, age, profession, weight and injury history. That's one reason why it's not simply a matter of cutting calories but a more involved process. Ideally if you can work with both a trainer and a nutritionist on a personalized program, you will put yourself in a great position to succeed.

Another "best practice" to success is to set up goals. Write them down. Repeat them every day. It's a pattern that highly successful people use and it's free! I love to set goals for myself. Make them a challenge, but make them attainable. Mix in a variety of short and long term goals. For instance if you're a size 16 maybe a long term goal is to fit into a size 12. Your short term goals, however, might be, lose 5 pounds, walk to work at least 2 times per week or join a swimming class. Reaching your short term goals is what keeps you going after and attaining your long-term goals.

Overall, when you lose weight too fast most likely you are losing muscle along with fat, and that's not what you want. When you lose "lean mass" that's bad for the tone and shape of your body, and also bad for your metabolism. Time, a targeted workout and clean diet will allow you to lose that fat forever. When I say forever, I am not promising the moon. I know some of you may be rolling your eyes, but nothing breeds success like success. When you change your life habits, eat better and lose the extra weight you want you will feel better about yourself. You'll have more energy and gained confidence not only in your looks but in accomplishing your goals.

2. I have an event coming up in 2 months. What's my best strategy for getting in better shape by then?

2 months is a reasonable period of time, and yet, in the same breath I must say it's not much time. You will need to be disciplined and follow your program. With such limited time, you can't fix everything, but I would pick 3 areas of focus that the client needs to work on, or 3 parts of her body that she feels are being judged when the spotlight is on her. For women, it's typically their arms, their waist, and their bottom. I tell my clients they can't hide behind sentences like "I was never good at that", or "I have these limits". This is the time to

set reasonable goals and push beyond your limits. And when you have that inevitable step back that challenges us all, don't let it turn you around. Move forward at the next opportunity.

It also helps to pick an activity that is right for you and fun to do. Think of a group of kids playing football or soccer. They are running, jumping, starting and stopping and having the time of their lives. Oh, and they're also exercising. Find your exercise in fun places. You'll stick with it longer and enjoy it more.

3. Is walking or running better for fat loss?

Here there is not a right or wrong answer. Running is definitely more efficient for fat loss than walking, but it's also very very tough on the body. If I had to chose one I would rather push most of you towards walking, power walking, and going up and down steps instead of running and risking knee issues or back pain. With walking you have to cover 1.5 times the distance you need to run to burn the same amount of calories, but I still feel it's a safe choice and a great lifestyle choice as well. Remember our goal is healthier bodies. I see no reason to put your body at risk of injury. Following a smart and safe regimen can get you into better shape and increase your level of fitness instead of decreasing it with an injury. Of course if running is your passion it fits under the category I spoke of earlier, do what you love.

4. Should I do cardio or weight training?

It shouldn't be an either or choice, it's like asking if you should eat only fruits or only vegetables. If you need to give priority to one style of workout however, weight training is like killing two birds with one stone and can give you benefits beyond building pure muscle mass. It tones your muscles and you burn more fat. Weight training bursts the metabolism which keeps you burning more calories even sitting in a chair 36 hours after your session. Also, the more lean muscle mass grows the more you burn. That's why men can usually eat more than a woman of the same weight. You will get a much better overall transformation doing weight work over cardio. If you've ever noticed someone who has lost a considerable amount of weight but looks somewhat soft, that is usually why. Yes they lost fat, but at the same time their muscles aren't toned and they don't give off the appearance we love and seek.

5. What are your recommended workouts for fast results?

I firmly believe that everyone of us is a different book, needing a different mix of cardio, weight training and other lifestyle changes for maximum benefit. With a tight deadline I like to alternate "Block training" and Pilates. Block Training allows you to reproduce an aerobic workout indoors without running or cycling. You will work the whole body changing the group of muscles to use every minute and also changing the posture and position of your body in space to target different aspects of the physiological training of the heart. The heart is a muscle after all! No props are needed with this type of training making it a great solution when traveling or when getting to the gym is not convenient

Basically, you would do 6 minutes of alternating work and 1 minute of stretching. For example: Triceps, Squats, Push ups, Rhomboids, Abs and Glutes all worked sequentially for 1 minute each, executed quickly and with no rest period between sections. This is followed immediately by 1 minute of stretching. Repeat this format with different muscle groups 4 to 5 times. At the end of the workout you will not only have accomplished a great calorie burn but added a good cardio workout and toned multiple muscle groups.

Pilates can be defined as "Strength and Stretch with control". It is a method I love and believe in and one in which I consistently see results. Pilates tones and strengthens the core muscles while keeping them long and lean. Most actions are executed in total range, always lengthening and moving, never stopping. This is one reason models and dancers love it, because they gain strength without the risk of bulking up their bodies. At the same time, lets not identify Pilates as a woman gentle stretching routine. Don't forget, Joseph Pilates moved to the United States to work with boxers and today we see basketball players and football players as well embracing this workout. Pilates can be a great compensatory workout used to achieve correct posture, rebalance our bodies and stay injury free. I see great results alternating block training with Pilates.

6. How can I speed up my recovery period?

Smart planning of your workout is the first key to managing your recovery period. By design, if you target alternate parts of the body and muscle groups you've given yourself a built in recovery period. Simply stated, If you work the upper limbs one day and the lower extremities the next, then each section is receiving the needed rest.

The real key to recovery, however, is Myofascial Stretching.

With this technique you don't only elongate the muscle but you put the fascia (connective tissue) in tension. The fascia connects the whole body, and the quality of our fascia helps determine our biological age and health. It's simplistic but imagine the fascia as a sophisticated bag that holds the muscle. When we want to change, strengthen or stretch the muscle you need to change the fascia first. That's why the normalization of the fascia through this specific type of stretching speeds up the recovery period between workouts.

7. How often should I workout?

To answer this question it's helpful to go back to the definition of periodization: the systematic planning of athletic or physical training. In periodization we formulate the relationship between time needed to reach a goal and frequency of working out. Let's see how this works with two different clients. If a client tells me that they have 2 months to get ready for a gala event, then clearly time is the priority. This goals timeline is not flexible so we will most likely have to work out 5 times a week. If however a client tells me they want to lose their post baby fat or define their arms we look at their lifestyle and focus on frequency. What can they commit to is the most important question.

8. How do I get a flat stomach?

Pilates. People often think doing crunches only will give them a six pack, forgetting that there is more to our midsection then just those muscles. The Obliques shape and thin the waistline while the transverse pulls the stomach flat. The abdominals need to be worked in all parts, and in different ranges of motion if we want a flat and strong stomach. Pilates works the stomach deeply and also teaches you how to connect the work and movement of your limbs to the core or center of your body. This allows you to learn how to exercise and instinctively use the abdominal muscles during your everyday life. The limb-core connection is also what helps you stay injury free: weights, loads and big movement are always supported by a strong core from where everything starts from.

9. How do I get rid of flabby arms?

Toned arms are important to women. Our evening dresses are often sleeveless and to look good you want not only toned triceps but also nicely toned shoulders. If I'm in a Pilates studio the arm chair or arm springs are great choices to tone my red carpet clients. The springs have an increasingly higher resistance that allows the muscles to work all points of action from the very start to the maximum extension without getting bulky, which is what many women are afraid of when working on their arms. While all muscles in the arm have their shaping importance I prioritize the triceps first. They are usually used the least in our everyday routines. I'll focus as well on the shoulders and back. The arms are connected to the back by many muscles like the inter-scapulae and lats, so by properly toning them you can achieve a healthy and toned look to your back, perfect for backless dresses as well. What really makes a difference for the gala event and beyond however is putting this all together. If in these 2 months you work to improve your posture, and pilates is great for that, that will exponentially increase the work you are doing on stomach and arms. It will act like a magnifying glass. You will stand taller, shoulders will look and be more relaxed, chest open, stomach lifted and flat... you will look better and radiate more confidence. The way we carry ourselves tells people about us. Men and women in all professions can benefit from this work and have an amazing return on their investment in training.

10. What short workouts can I do between work?

When your schedule get busier then expected you need to have a plan B ready. Short workouts that you can execute at home or in your office can save you. For example, you can exercise your upper back muscles almost anywhere by lying on your stomach and lifting the arms up doing flies. You can work the triceps by doing dips using the office chair or couch. Arm reinforcement can be done using bottle of water or push ups, either inclined using a table or a desk or flat on the floor. Decide to commit to take the stairs when you get on the subway and up and down to your office. If you are located at a low floor you can always go all the way up to the 10th floor and then back down to your floor and add repetitions as you get more fit. These are only a few examples. When time gets short the biggest risk you have to your workout routine is not doing it. When you get creative and squeeze in a short workout, even if it's not ideal it keeps the momentum going and you feel good about yourself.

11. What is the best diet to follow?

There are many diets out there, some better than others but I don't feel like giving names because it's not a one choice fits all answer. The most important thing is to seek out the freshest organic, non-GMO fruits and vegetables available. Look for grass fed meats and wild seafood. A nutrition plan needs to contain proteins to lower blood sugar, carbs to raise blood sugar and fats to help normalize blood sugar. This is why it's so important to always combine them in every meal.

The other major factor with diet is a lifestyle. Stress causes cortisol release and the storage of fat around the midsection. When talking weight loss, you must look for ways to lower stress and increase the quantity and quality of your sleep routine.

Also, don't forget about water. Why? Because water keeps us young, is the best and least expensive health and beauty remedy we can find. In a workout and diet regimen like I'm suggesting, the hydrating and purifying action of water is very important. All the waste we accumulate in our bodies is released faster and more efficiently thanks to the acceleration and improvement in the physiological processes brought on by water intake. Water also hydrates the fascia which is a key to good health. As a general rule drink at least 2 liters of water a day though that varies by the activity level, season, food intake and other fluids ingested. Coffee for instance dehydrates the body, that means if you like to drink coffee you'll have to increase your water intake. I suggest you drink from clear water bottles. Drinking water by the bottle makes it easier to track your intake and the clear bottle is a reminder of what's left for you to finish to reach your goals.

12. Do I need to take dietary supplements?

In case of any deficiency, supplements can help, however, if one is eating high-quality food and making healthy choices supplements should not be necessary.

13. What tips do you have for healthy food on the go?

Snacks and meals on the go should follow the same rules and principles outlined in our diet regimen. Try to be consistent mixing proteins, carbs and fats at each snack. Try to avoid extremes. Eating too much before a workout will make you sleepy and slow while not eating enough can make you dizzy. In either event you won't be at your efficient best.

14. Who is your ideal client to work with?

The client who commits! If there are trust and commitment, everything is possible and results will be easier to achieve. You need to stick to a program and give it a chance. It's not productive to select bits and pieces of the latest fad like your picking chocolates out of a box. Trust your professional trainer and ask questions, but then do the work with passion and commitment.

15. What are the main benefits of working with a personal trainer?

Your trainer should be your partner, as invested in your results as you are. That means listening to your goals and moving you at a safe and steady pace. Motivating you when you need it, and pulling back when you are at your limits.

The main benefit for clients is they don't need to stress over what is right to do, what they should do or how far they should push themselves today. All those decisions are handled by a person they trust. That is not to say they simply follow instructions and walk through a military repetition of exercises. While I make the decisions, a committed client is fully engaged and actively participates in the process.

The other main benefit of working with a trainer is results. It's like trying to learn a language by computer or "one on one" with a language teacher. The only difference is if you mispronounce a word working with a computer it doesn't hurt as much as when you overdo a workout you saw on Youtube.

A trainer also makes your gym membership worthwhile because you actually end up using it instead of forgetting you have one.

Please tell us how readers can get in contact with you here:

Website: ilariaCavagna.com

Email: ilaria917@gmail.com

Phone: +1 917 770 4065

Linkedin: Ilaria Cavagna

Facebook: ilaria Cavagna

Twitter: @ilariacavagna

Instagram: ilariacavagna

CHAPTER 13

CLIFFORD JOSEPH

Please tell us about your company here:

Fitness-Essentials.net is a company that offers Fitness & Nutrition Life Coaching in person or via video chat/phone. Our goal is helping people understand body mechanics and proper movement patterns for better muscle recruitment which results in a longer training life with minimal injury in addition to getting the desired results. Our methods are to push your limit, challenge your thought process and find your reason why which we believe will keep you motivated during the times where you are at your weakest. Whether it's body composition, meditation, decreasing stress levels or overcoming an illness or injury that caused muscle atrophy our fitness & nutritional life coaches are driven to help you meet and exceed your goals. We consult and design fitness floors for companies, organizations and communities who are looking to improve or create a health space for their occupancies. We look to create innovative fitness floors that will help increase proper movement patterns, enhance proper body mechanics, and incorporate functional movement.

1. What is the best way to lose fat?

The best way to lose fat is to build muscle. First thing everyone needs to understanding is there's a difference between overall weight, body fat percentage and BMI. In addition to that learning more about your resting metabolic rate(RMR) will help you find out what the best ways to lose fat. 1lb of muscle will continue to burn energy even while you're sleeping and although it's not a huge number of caloric energy it's better than not burning any energy at rest.

Many people I have encountered believed that doing cardio all the time would help them lose the fat, the fact is doing all types of cardiovascular exercises actually works your circulatory system home of vital organs the lymphatic system which allows fluids and nutrients to pass to and from the body in addition to regulating hormones and pH . It's great to burn the maximum amount of calories you can while working on a bike, stairmaster, treadmill or elliptical just know that once you stop working your cardiovascular system(also known as the circulatory system) you stop burning calories and depending on your speed and Intensity you could be missing your fat storage and instead be burning sugars which will defeat the purpose of burning fat. Building muscle with a solid program will gain great results and your body composition will change which mean your waistline will change.

In addition to that when you are training with resistance and building muscle you will keep burning calories hours after you have left the gym. When your body repairs itself, you need to burn energy (calories) in order to heal the muscle. Men and women can build muscle and look great and get amazing results while burning more energy with every pound added, So go out and burn that fat by building some muscle! A solid program with resistance training and cardio is key to getting great results.

2. I have an event coming up in 2 months. What's my best strategy for getting in better shape by then?

2 months is 8 weeks so you must first know what your goal is, if it's weight loss you will be considering a more vigorous

workout which will consist of cardio and resistance training 5 times a week in addition to a yoga class and flexibility program your body will need at least 24 - 48 hours to recover so use the steam room and the sona to remove toxin from the body while you're resting.

Program design is key when looking to get the maximum amount of results in a shortened time period think about swimming or long walks on days you're not in the gym to keep burning as many energy. Let's keep in mind no matter how much you are moving if you're not paying attention to your nutrition you won't be happy at the end of the 8-week program.

Nutrition is one of the pillars in losing weight quickly and efficiently there are so many diets and fads out there that will challenge you to only eat the minimal amount of food in order to lose weight. I don't like nor do I believe that fad diets are the way to go and this is why, fad diets work for some people temporarily, but most of them have an expiration date after the expiration date people don't have the same accountability therefore they can have a weight gain response. You need to know what your body burns while you at rest (RMR), how many calories do you burn on a daily basis.

After finding that out either speak with a nutritionist or cut out some of the non essentials like beers and wine, sodas and sugar-filled drinks. Your body need to focus on processing fat as energy and not be distracted by sugar or alcohol, Once you know how much calories you are burning on a daily basis you need to go to the gym or park and burn off least 1,000 calories a day every day until your event and not eat any more than what your body is using at rest to life off of. For example, if at rest you are burning 1,500 calories then you need to burn 1,000 calories during your exercise program in order to see the desired results. You will be using 1,500 calories a day to function so make sure those are high in nutritional values, high protein for muscle growth and maintenance as well as healthy fats and carbohydrates from veggies.

It's not about starving yourself for two months it's about being able to maintain your new eating habits for life and seeing the results of your new program in 2 months will not only have you ready for this event but others down the line as well. Be proactive and be prepared for your healthy figure. If you're looking to put on some muscle before your event, you still need to know how many calories you're burning at rest (RMR).

From there proper nutrition and resistance training will be key. Most of us don't have time to hit the gym twice a day but for those looking for amazing results and who want to build muscle that can be a good game plan. If you are hitting the gym twice a day program design will be critical so you don't over train your body and injure yourself, flexibility training will be a huge part of your program and getting into some type of yoga class should be a part of that twice a day program at least twice a week.

Know what your body fat is before your two-month event starts so that you can enjoy the results after you're done making great gains. In both cases you will need a rest day because your body needs to recover so enjoy your Sunday off by the pool, make sure you are getting at least seven hours of sleep a day and don't stress your body out before your workouts or you will store fat in your gut. Keep these tips in mind and you will be on your way to a great look during your event!

3. Is walking or running better for fat loss?

This is all about knowing your Active Metabolic Rate (AMR) or Zone Training which has been popping up everywhere, some people live by it others don't believe in it. The fact is our body burns two types of energy sources one being Fat and the other Carbohydrates. Fat is a slow burning fuel similar to burning coal it takes a while to start up and once its going it will burn for hours whereas Carbohydrates (sugars) burn like lighter fuel which means it goes up fast and burns faster. Simple right well not exactly.. if you are walking at a low heart rate like walking your dog or strolling with your friends down 5th ave New York as your head to work; although you are burning energy while you're moving if this is something you do everyday than your body will plateau and you will stop seeing the results of fat loss and instead be in a maintenance period where you may not see change at all. Our bodies are the best adaptors on the planet and because of that we need to think of all the variables that comes with training the body to lose fat and gain muscle. I suggest if you don't run or walk start with walking and use an activity tracker shot for 10,000 steps a day this will help you keep track and in 6 to 8 weeks you will need to create a change so that your body needs to adapt once again. Either change your route from flat to hills or add some stairs even jog a few of those steps this will keep your body excited and it will need to meet the demands by burning more energy. If you're not killing yourself meaning sprinting at a very high heart rate you will burn fat. Once you are sprinting at a high heart rate you turn off your fat energy and go into the carbohydrates for the extra boost of energy. This isn't a bad thing in fact its great for your heart and lunges to push to those high heart rate zones. The Circulatory system will get stronger and the muscles responsible for working will tighter(in shape), Once you are able to walk and jog at then start doing interval training another great variable if you are a walker and are just getting into running. I like to tell my clients to look at our olympic sprinters, hurdlers and cross country runners body types, our muscles are made of slow twitch and fast twitch fibers and depending on what you're looking for you can see the results within these different competitors. Our sprinters and hurdlers are interval runners where they are walking and sprinting in addition to training with resistance meanwhile our cross country runners are slow and steady and burning a massive amount of fat. These athletes are at the peak of fitness and there body fat percentage is extremely low on both ends but you can see from this example how zone training does play a major role in our metabolic fitness and cardio is important in our overall health.

4. Should I do cardio or weight training?

You should do both! We have three major systems in the body, the skeletal system, muscular system and circulatory system and they all need to be trained. We live in a much different world than our forefathers, we are not hunters and gatherers and we don't need to walk miles for water or food. In some country where that is still the norm you can see how muscular and healthy people are, most live very long lives and have the ability to run and play well in there 70's. The body adapts and sometimes when you have chairs in air conditioned offices your body gets softer and weaker do to the conditions it is accustomed to. The circulatory system has a huge responsibility without it we wouldn't have proper hormone balance, we wouldn't get fluids to and from different areas of the body and our heart, lunges and other organs that are apart of the circulatory system wouldn't be strong enough for us to do daily tasks. Doing cardio its a key part of a health way of life so go out and play, jump rope or just push your small child in the stroller up and down the street cardio is here to stay. Weight training is huge as I said before building muscle burns calories the more muscle you have the small your fat cells become and any extra energy burned while you sleep is welcome, resistance training gives you strong bones and helps develop body composition. We will pick things up and put them down most of our lives and weight training helps us do that. A good program will make sure that when you are picking things up and putting them down your body is doing it functionally and recruiting the right muscle to complete the task. Any good program will have a balance of Cardio, Weight (Resistance) Training and Flexibility Training.

5. What are your recommended workouts for fast results?

Fast results is a relative term, If you have a lot of weight to lose and you're just starting your program than just committing yourself to a stabilization and cardio program will get you great results for your first 6 to 8 weeks. If you are a long time gym rat and you are looking for fast result you may need to look at your program design and find out if there has been enough variables. If you have been doing the same bench press for years you may need to change it up meaning use dumbbells and a stability ball to create a super set. Changing the exercises routine and creating more stability has proven to show up in the amount people can lift and in our body composition. Vertical loading is another great way to challenge the body, instead of doing one muscle group a day do all the muscle groups. Think about your program whether you're just starting out or if you have been training a long time and find ways to challenge the body while maintaining great form and proper postural alignment. With great form comes great responsibility to maintain it during movement.

There are many different ways to change the program design in order to see great results whether it's weight lose, weight gain or better posture if you know where you started you can be impressed with where you end up in a few short weeks.

6. How can I speed up my recovery period?

There are some great supplements that can help with a speedy recovery, Fish Oil, Turmeric, Curcumin, and high quality protein are a few things that can help with repairing the muscle and keeping down the inflammation. The key to a quick recovery is limiting how much inflammation is in the body after a workout. Sleep is one of the best ways to naturally recover and should be a key part of your program in addition to foam rolling and proper stretching after workouts and before workouts. Dynamic stretching before getting into the routine can get the mind and body prepared for the workout while a foam rolling and static stretch and release toxins and inflammation into the bloodstream to be processed out of the body. Drink water 128 ounces a day will keep your hydrated and feeling focused and add multivitamins to your supplements in order to get your daily dose of nutrients.

7. How often should I workout?

If you are looking to see change and I mean any change at all and you're new to the gym than you need to workout a minimum of 2 times a week if you are doing anything less you will not train your body to change. Our body needs a routine in order to recognize that it's time to change its old habits a minimum of 2 hours of resistance training a week can start to get your body aware that it's time to mobilize the fat that has been stored up for years and use that energy in order to meet the demands of your new routine. If you are looking for more results than you can add days into it, you should also do at least 7,500 steps a day. We sit way too much as a society and because of that our body starts to shut off muscles that we otherwise need in life, as we get older we feel this in chronic pain, muscle imbalance, bad posture which leads to hormone imbalance and improper organ functions to name a few things that occur therefore move your body and enjoy the world outside of the office and/or home.

8. How do I get a flat stomach?

It's not just crunches and planks that will get your stomach flat, your nutrition is a big part of what will get you there. cardio and resistance training will be a major part of this program although our body determines where we will lose fat first before our mind and our will. We can't just say I want to lose fat in my stomach and poof it's flat after a few weeks. A huge part of stomach fat is stress levels if you are very stressed out at work and/or home you will store a huge amount of fat in your abdomen. Another thing to look at is cortisol levels it helps the body use sugar and/or fat for energy as well as manage stress. Cortisol levels can be affected by many things, such as physical or emotional stress, strenuous activity, infection, or injury. Cortisol level may show problems with the adrenal glands or pituitary gland it also release a hormone called adrenocorticotropic hormone (ACTH) when this is in balance our body will operate normal we sleep at night and wake up in the morning with energy to take on the day when it's out of wake our body will want to crash mid afternoon our stress levels will be all over the place and we can not focus. This affects our workouts as well because while we train we add more stress to the body and if the body is overstressed it will store fat in our abdomen causing the opposite effects. It's important to know what going on inside the body as well as outside of it in order to get the results desired. Learning about how your pituitary gland and adrenal gland manages the hormones in your body will be a key tool in losing stomach fat. Get your hormones in balance.

9. How do I get rid of flabby arms?

This is easy get more muscle! building muscle in the upper body is a great way to get rid of flabby arms. Most people don't realize that our arms are needed to do all our upper body movements whether we are working our chest or our back we need to use our arms as secondary movers in order to push and pull the resistance around. Isolating the arms are also a great way to get them in shape, and even in your planks and cobras you use your arms to stabilize your shoulders in order to focus on pulling in your stomach. In your program don't just think about Isolating your arms think about all the ways you can use them in order to move the resistance around and go for it. With the right coach, you should be seeing those arms tighten up after a few weeks.

10. What short workouts can I do between work?

The best ways I feel to get a quick or short workout in between work is to use your environment as your gym. It's not always convenient to get to the gym between lunch hours because of showering and changing but 15 minutes a day is still better than nothing at all. If you don't have a place close enough to you make sure you park the car in the furthest place you can from the building and walk to it and back to the office. Do you have a staircase? Use the steps in between lunch and do a few laps up and down them to see how far you can get. How about a office space? You can bring in a mat and a stability ball into your office and practice some of those core movements you're trying to master. Do you have a beautiful outdoor space? take a stroll around the complex and bring a co- worker with you. If you look at your environment as a playground, you can have so much fun just playing around with friends and getting a great workout in. It's team building and will help get you the results you're looking for. 15 minute workout routines that only require a TRX resistance bands or tubes that can easily be packed into a backpack or stored in a desk is a great way to get a total body workout in, think about it your have two set and 25 reps of TRX chest press, rows, squats, lunges, rear delt pulls, planks, knee tucks, and hamstring curls. After that workout, you may need to pack a change of clothes.

11. What is the best diet to follow?

The best diet to follow is the one you can stick with for the rest of your life. If you are unable to eat the same thing every day then that won't work for you will it? You need to customize your diet and find what will work with your lifestyle and then commit to it. I have found that for people who are working out three to five times a week a higher protein diet helps get great results because they retain the muscle and they're satisfied with their meals. Everyone is different and we all have different reactions to foods so learn what your body is sensitive to and remove it from your diet, alcohol can be a big sabotage to any diet plan don't just think about what you're eating but also keep in mind what you're drinking. Diet drinks have a lot of chemicals in them that do negative things to the body and processed foods although its proteins can be detrimental to our overall health don't overwork your liver and kidneys by eating and drinking processed diet food find healthy Non-Genetically Modified Organisims (GMO) organic and grass feed food to eat and drink learn what your Resting Metabolic Rate is and eat what's needed while burning off the energy through a great workout program .

12. Do I need to take dietary supplements?

Supplements are an important part of a nutrition program, if you are trying to lose weight there is no way you can eat all the nutrients needed in order to get the results needed and not go over on your daily caloric intake. We need to focus on keeping your calories down while we are in that stage of training. If we are trying to build muscle for gains than keeping down the inflammation in order to recover will require supplementation. There is a key thing to know about supplements and that is know that what the ingredients are in the bottle have been looked at by a third party pharmacy. Look for third-party providers on the labels of the supplements you take so you know that someone has checked it out, you don't want to take one multivitamin that has double the dose and another that doesn't have the required amount. Also recognized the advised requirements is created for the perfect individual as if they're in a bubble you may need more or less depending on your goals. Find a nutritionist who can help you customize your supplementation and nutrition in order for them to work together to get the desired results.

13. What tips do you have for healthy food on the go?

The best tips for healthy snacks on the go are the ones you can pre-pack. High protein snacks are great they will keep you feeling full for a longer period of time between meals. Pack things like boiled eggs, Nuts and cheese, fruits are alright but can be high in sugar and cause you to become hungry after a couple hours so add something that has high protein and a healthy fat such as avocado or almond butter. If you're stuck on the road and you have nothing to eat and you have to stop at a fast food place avoid the process food which is everything on the menu. Since everything has calories now you can avoid the landmines (burgers and fries) by choosing smaller meals like wraps or salads. Be aware of your week and plan ahead if you're truly trying to do better with you results then this is another major part of your program that you will focus on. Remember your nutrition is 70% of the plan and if it's off you will have a hard time getting the desired results.

14. Who is your ideal client to work with?

I enjoy working with anyone who is willing to learn and not afraid of change, my motto is embraced the change. Your body, your mind, and your spirit will change for the better if you are willing to embrace it and not plateau in life. I have had the pleasure to work with kids just starting their fitness journey as well as seniors learning new ways in which to activate muscles that they thought would not work due to age. I have worked with clients after they have finished a Physical Therapy session and need continued training and clients who are looking to be the best most explosive athletes in their sport. If you have an open mind and are willing to challenge yourself, I will be honored to coach you!

15. What are the main benefits of working with a personal trainer?

I believe that the benefits of working with a fitness professional is the education that they can and should provide to their clients. We have mechanics that we go to for car service and doctors we go to for health concerns after discovering we are ill. A great fitness professional should be in the preventive health business, what I mean by that is personal trainers are helping people understand muscle dysfunction in order to help avoid injury in addition the education of the fitness professional should be given to the client during every session therefore allowing the client to be more educated on their individual needs. Whether it's correcting posture that could help with hormone imbalances or learning how to correct muscle imbalances in order to contract the proper muscle during corrective exercise programing the fitness professional get to help people before the injuries and illnesses occur. And in some causes help with removing the accumulative injury all together when correcting improper movement patterns.

Program design and teaching about the variables in a training program is another value that a client can get from working with a fitness professional, there will be hours of focus time dedicated to creating the most effective program for a client and that client get the benefit of a completed and dedicated workout every time they hit the workout floor.

Proper lifting techniques are among the biggest benefits for clients, just pushing weights around and not truly understand how the muscle group works can cause muscle imbalances and which can lead a client into an accumulative injuries cycle, a fitness professionals continued education (which is necessary in order to stay certified personal trainers) are always learning which trickles down to the clients always getting the latest in education from our industries finest. Power lifts need to be performed with proper posture and kinetic chain alignment and sometimes you just can't tell if you're doing something right that's when having another set of eyes that knows what to look for and how to cue you to lift properly can be a huge advantage.

Finally motivation and accountability to get to the gym on a scheduled time and make that the most exciting and productive part of your day for your personal goals. This time isn't about your employer's, employees or your clients, you're not concerned with your husband or wife or kids. It's about how you're getting stronger. Every hour it's about what you need to do for your mental, physical and emotional growth. It's that great feeling of accomplishment after a hard hour that makes you feel you can take on all of life's obstacles and crush them. Having a coach that cares about you just as much as you care about yourself is key to obtaining your desired results and a one on one or small group session with someone who will be there with you through your journey cheering you on and pushing your limits will always be an invaluable tool to use during your training life.

Please tell us how readers can get in contact with you here:

Website: http: //www.fitness-essentials.net

Please feel free to contact me via email cj@fitness-essentials. net and/or info@fitness-essentials.net

For any reason emails bounce back you can also reach me at cliff.o.joseph@gmail.com

CONCLUSION

The power to change the way you look and feel about yourself is truly in your hands. While this book is mainly about getting into shape for an upcoming event, our hope is that you continue to maintain a healthy lifestyle even beyond that. Do what you need to in order to keep to your health goals. It is a journey that is well worth it!

www.ingramcontent.com/pod-product-compliance
Lightning Source LLC
Chambersburg PA
CBHW060357290526
45791CB00002B/540